HYGGE

Practical Step-by-step Guide to a Cosy & Simple
Lifestyle

(A Danish Concept of Cosy and Simple Living)

Gwendolyn Tucker

Published by Kevin Dennis

Gwendolyn Tucker

All Rights Reserved

Hygge: Practical Step-by-step Guide to a Cosy & Simple
Lifestyle (A Danish Concept of Cosy and Simple Living)

ISBN 978-1-989965-79-5

Legal & Disclaimer

The information contained in this book is not designed to replace or take the place of any form of medicine or professional medical advice. The information in this book has been provided for educational and entertainment purposes only.

The information contained in this book has been compiled from sources deemed reliable, and it is accurate to the best of the Author's knowledge; however, the Author cannot guarantee its accuracy and validity and cannot be held liable for any errors or omissions. Changes are periodically made to this book. You must consult your doctor or get professional medical advice before using any of the suggested remedies, techniques, or information in this book.

Upon using the information contained in this book, you agree to hold harmless the Author from and against any damages, costs, and expenses, including any legal fees potentially resulting from the application of any of the information provided by this guide. This disclaimer applies to any damages or injury caused by the use and application, whether directly or indirectly, of any advice or information presented, whether for breach of contract, tort, negligence, personal injury, criminal intent, or under any other cause of action.

You agree to accept all risks of using the information presented inside this book. You need to consult a professional medical practitioner in order to ensure you are both able and healthy enough to participate in this program.

Table of Contents

Introduction

It's true that most people live hectic lives. We've become accustomed to instant gratification. But, this increases the stress we place ourselves under. There's stress to keep up with your neighbors, to do better at work, and even to make sure the customers you serve have what they need, instantly.

There is little doubt that the pandemic has affected everyone, life may never be the same again. But, just as there is numerous hardships to face in the coming months and years, there is also an opportunity to start again.

Of course, most people can't simply change their lifestyle or walk away from everything. You have commitments that need to be fulfilled, people to look after, and a life to live!

But, the current crisis does provide the opportunity to re-evaluate what is important and what you want from the future.

It's probably not the same thing that you wanted a few months ago. In fact, many people are looking for a way to improve their work/life balance and make the most of the time they have available.

It has led to a great interest in alternate lifestyles. There are many to choose from, nomadic hippies, running organic farms, taking up yoga, heading to a Buddhist, or another religious retreat. Unfortunately, as mentioned, it's not possible for most people to simply give up their current life. This is where Hygge steps in.

Hygge is not a new lifestyle concept. In fact, it is one of the simplest and oldest concepts. Best of all, it's something that you can do alongside your current life. You simply need to understand the concept and embrace the ordinary moments that are so often overlooked.

Take a stroll through the following pages to understand the origins of Hygge, what it really is, and how you can apply it to your life.

It doesn't matter what age you are, you can embrace Hygge and adopt a new outlook on life.

Chapter 1: The Science Of Happiness

It's human nature to want to be happy, and cultures across the world have their own ways to pursue happiness, claim it, and then express it. And while happiness does exist in all cultures, its meaning and expression vary significantly. Yet, despite these differences, happy people do seem to have different habits and viewpoints than others who are miserable.

For starters, happiness for most people comes from experiences rather than from material gain. Yes, money is an awesome motivator on some level, and will probably yield a great deal of pleasure momentarily. But that pleasure is often short-lived, and too often confused with happiness. Once things go back to normal and pleasure subsides, or say, you get used to the money, the happiness seems to level out as well.

People who are not happy with what they have believe that they'll be happier when they get what they want. For instance, when someone gets a large house with a swimming pool or gets a promotion they've been chasing for a long time, they are momentarily happy. But the problem is that once they get used to their new belongings or status in life, in time they return back to their pre-existing state of happiness or unhappiness whichever the case may be.

On the other hand, happy people invest more in their experiences than anything else. Science reveals that happy people show specific ways of thinking and acting which strongly impact their sense of happiness and peace of mind. And while there are many habits, here are some of the most prominent that distinguishes happy people from others who aren't so happy.

Relationships

People with one or more close friendships are significantly happier than others who don't. It doesn't really matter if there's a broad network of close relationships or not, but what seems relevant is how often someone participates or cooperates in activities. This frequency of participation gives people a chance to share their personal feelings with a close friend or family member.

The benefit that impacts happiness from relationships comes from different capacities and for different reasons. For instance, successful relationships, whether romantic or platonic, increases a person's emotional well-being, creates stability, teaches them how to be a good friend and gives them someone to count on and trust in times of need. Relationships also give people someone to vent to in the face of challenges. Each type of relationship elicits different responses that help people grow and learn more about themselves.

Acts of kindness

Another aspect of happiness shows that people who care for others or volunteer on a regular basis appear to be more content, happier and even less depressed. 'Caring' is a rather broad term for it can involve volunteering with a club or organized group, where you may donate your time or money. Or it may imply reaching out to a peer or colleague who seems to be struggling. It could even be something as simple as helping an elderly person cross the road or help someone get something off the shelf at the grocery store.

Most people who care for others in a selfless manner do so out of a genuine desire to help and improve the world around them. However, contemporary research has shown that caring has benefits for everyone involved. For instance, people who volunteer or assist others on a frequent basis tend to present higher psychological well-being. This includes fewer depressive symptoms and a higher degree of life satisfaction. Reaching out like this shows improved well-being and a positive effect on others.

Spiritual engagement and meaning

Studies show a close association between spirituality and happiness. Spirituality emphasizes greater meaning in life as it provides people a chance to engage in a meditative act. Meditation also links strongly with wellbeing because it can calm the body, reduce stress and anxiety, and also support positive thinking.

The practice of revered moments in everyday life whether it is journal writing or practicing spiritual exercises has been linked to reduced stress levels and increased psychological wellbeing. Also, spirituality can help provide people with hope, perspective and a deeper sense of meaning. When people believe in something higher than themselves, it helps them stay optimistic in trying times, and this fosters resilience as a coping mechanism.

Positive mindset

People who are happy often hold gratitude, hope, and mindfulness dear. Grateful people also demonstrate more positive emotion, higher satisfaction, and a lower rate of stress and depression. And when you are grateful for every little thing you have, or every little experience you go through, you don't tend to chase after material things or gains. Instead, whatever you have in your life at that moment is enough to gratify you and make you happy.

Positive mindset, or optimism, by itself offers many health benefits such as improving the immune system, preventing chronic disease, and helping people cope with unfortunate news. When optimism is paired with gratitude, it makes grateful people happier, receive more social support, be less stressed, and less depressed.

Along with these few, happy people also take care of their physical health and exercise regularly. They tend to find their flow, meaning they engage in activities they enjoy immensely. This is typically something that brings them intrinsic motivation and uses their strengths, whatever they may be, for a purpose greater than their own personal goals.

Now, if you look at all these traits carefully, you'll come to realize that these are all experiences. Garnering and fostering relationships is an experience, engaging in kind acts is an experience, and so is practicing spiritual engagement. These experiences get preserved as memories which stay with us for a long time and so the more happy memories you have to cherish, the cozier and more comfortable your life becomes.

Another thing to consider here is that happiness also brings relief. It may be relief from stress which can escalate easily when activities, which are otherwise mildly stressful, start to feel overwhelming. As someone experiences too much stress in their life, relief in these instances can overtime add up to increase resilience.

Doing little things to uplift your mood can really have a long-term effect on resilience against stress. Every time you engage in a pleasant act, you take a step towards feeling less stress in the present as well as in the future. This gesture also lets you enjoy other perks as well.

For instance, it's said a good mood leads to more resources. Resources here refer to making connections with people. When you express positive emotions, you strengthen your social connections because you seem cordial. People won't shy away from approaching you which can lead to solid friendships, reliable colleagues, and happy bosses.

On the other hand, demonstrating a negative state of emotion can cause you to develop monomania where you fixate excessively on the adverse that you bypass good opportunities in your life. But those who stay happy are more likely develop personal resources which are allied with resilience towards stress.

These stress-busting resources come in many forms. For instance, first and foremost, you have personal resilience. Then there is interpersonal resilience in the form of supportive friends. Finally, practical resilience can manifest itself as secure financial standing. This upturn in resources brings about more recurrent happy moods, and creates an upward spiral. This, in turn, improves your health, increases your happiness, and boosts your life satisfaction.

As we move further into this book, you'll see how being a happy person will help you embrace hygge easier. Relationships, graciousness, mindfulness, and optimism run high in a hygge setting. If you already have these positive traits in your lifestyle, hygge may not be such a major transition as you imagine it to be.

Chapter 2: What Is The Meaning Of Hygge

Hygge is a Danish and Norwegian language noun used to define a feeling, a social atmosphere, an action related to a sense of comfort, security, welcome and familiarity. It expresses a concept similar to the German word Gemütlichkeit.

The concept of hygge is not aimed at the pursuit of momentary happiness, but at everyday happiness, which contributes to a sense of fulfilment in the long term.

Hygge must instill a pleasant feeling and feeling good is the main priority. Hygge helps you to experience exactly a feeling day by day.

According to an EU survey, Danish citizens are the happiest in the world, as they spend more time with family and friends and feel more relaxed than others feel.

To be hyggeligt (an adjective derived from hygge) you need to focus on the simple things that make you feel good, recreating a welcoming environment where you can fully enjoy the daily pleasures that life offers.

Typical hyggeligt activities are for example: expressing oneself freely, moving away from everyday life commitments, and sharing food by baking cakes, cookies, bread for guests and neighbors.

The exact opposite is "unhyggeligt".

What is Hygge

It is especially about achieving a state of happiness and satisfaction that goes beyond just feeling happy.

Those who are hyggeligt can rejoice in life's little things and enjoy time together with their friends.

The hyggeligt person transforms their home into a place of well-being.

Being hyggeligt does not cost anything. To be hygge you do not need to spend. It is about being happy with yourself, enjoying the moment and leaving negative thoughts behind.

When you become a hygge, you will be able to enjoy the moment and appreciate the small things in your daily life.

Enjoying the things we have like nature, for example, belongs to the hygge.

This Danish way of life is mainly based on cutting down on our hectic everyday life.

The hygge teaches you to listen to your inner self again, look inside yourself and recognize what you really need.

The three elements to live Hyggeligt

The hygge experience is based on three fundamental elements: interiority, contrast and atmosphere.

Interiority

In the hygge, you can distinguish between the inner and outer space. Interiority is the ability to recognize oneself as a well-defined presence, which exists in relation to others, the place and the passage of time. When we practice hygge, we are aware that our refuge has physical and temporal boundaries. Hygge comes from a culture that gives value to the concept of inner space. Mind, home and country are the insides of the hygge.

Contrast

When we practice hygge, we establish a sense of distance between us and the rest of the world, a contrast between the feeling of being in a moment of pleasure and the awareness that life around us continues to flow.

This contrast is perceived through the emphasis on spatial, temporal and social conditions. Example, day versus night, shelter versus exposure, light versus shade, interior versus exterior, heat versus cold, relaxation versus work, immobility versus activity, peace versus conflict.

Atmosphere

The atmosphere is the third element of the hygge, which means creating a feeling of warmth, a harmonious environment, a sense of fulfillment. We will discuss this concept in more detail in chapter 5.

Chapter 3: Ten Spring Hygge Tips

Spring is one of the most beautiful times of the year with blooming flowers and longer days of sunlight. It is the rebirth of nature leaving behind the harsh winter and reminding us that life is a series of beginnings. Practicing the art of Hygge in the spring is not a difficult task. And if you are in fact just starting the journey, there is no better time than spring. The following tips may be ideas for you to incorporate into a Hygge experience.

Bring fresh flowers into your home on a weekly basis and place them in your favorite vase. If you cannot pick them from your own flower garden, then stop by your local market. Tulips, daffodils, or hyacinths are perfect in the spring. Use a vase that is special to you or one that will introduce a moment of nostalgia. Fresh flowers are good any time of year, but spring flowers will push away those winter blues, and let everyone in your household know that a change is coming in the form of Hygge.

Clip stems from apple, cherry, plum, or pear trees. Place them in a vase of warm water, and before long, they will start to bloom. They are beautiful and smell delightful. They will probably not bear fruit, but have some of that fruit handy in a fruit basket near your trimming.

Switch up your bedding. Take off any heavy bed linens and replace with soft light cotton. You may even want to take down any heavy or dark drapes and lighten up your window coverings. This will also lighten up the atmosphere in your home and invite a more positive attitude into the space. Our surroundings, especially color, can play a part in setting a tone or mood for our homes; for example, blues are the most calming and muted dusty shades of other colors are as well. In Feng Shui, colors are used to bring different energies into the home such as passionate red, energetic yellow, or restorative green.

Replace that morning coffee with green tea, herbal tea, or a selection of juices. Go out on a limb, and try tropical juices that bring the Caribbean into your kitchen. The "no problem man" environment will welcome a more relaxed attitude. Put on a little reggae music and forget about work, school, or soccer practice for a few minutes. Mornings are normally the place the mood for the day begins, so mix it up, and make mornings more mysterious and surprising for your family. Don't do the same old things or make the same menu for breakfast. Create a moment of anticipation for your family, so they are excited about rolling out of bed.

Set out a couple of bird feeders or bird baths in a place where they can be viewed while you and your family enjoy breakfast or when you pull up a lawn chair on your deck or patio. Watching the different species of birds and even those pesky squirrels can be a Hygge moment. Humming birds are very entertaining, and they encompass the miracle that is nature.

The spring rains are beautiful in most cases and bring a cleansing to the earth. Open up the windows and let the fresh smell of the rain infiltrate your house. Turn off the television for a period, and listen as the rain drops fall onto the roof. There is nothing more relaxing and Hygge than welcoming the spring rains.

Sometimes spring bring some gusty winds, especially near the coast. Go to a local toy or hobby store and pick out a kite. Who would think that a piece of cloth connected to a string in the hands of a child could bring so many smiles and happiness to a family? Young and old experience a sense of wonder and peace while gazing into the sky at a beautiful colorful kite. I would avoid the kites with skull and crossbones or witches, if you want a Hygge kite experience. Flying kites in the park on a windy day is not only enjoyable, but Hygge is its purest sense.

Decorate your dining room table to welcome springtime. Use colored hollowed out eggs, flowers, pastel colored candles, napkins, or vines common to your area. There are many stores that have these items, and they are usually very inexpensive.

Pick up an outdoor game at the store such as corn hole, bocce ball, badminton, or horseshoes. Make some lemonade or a refreshing adult beverage and enjoy the game with your mate, family, or friends. I would not overly emphasize the competition aspect of the game with rewards, but everyone loves to win, and there is nothing we can do about human nature. Is winning Hygge? Well, probably only to the winner.

Remove all clutter from your kitchen or bathroom. Replace with fresh items such as spring smelling candles, bowl of lemons or limes, and new refreshing soaps. A single flower will also create a Hygge moment. Also, replace kitchen and bath towels with lighter spring like colors.

Spring itself ushers in a wonderful sense of Hygge each year. Nature reminds us that we must stop and enjoy the colors, and scents of a new beginning. If you want to practice the art of Hygge, simply bring the outside... inside.

Chapter 4: Using Hygge In Your Life

People enjoy feeling cozy, happy, and peaceful, and you do not have to move to Denmark if you want to embrace this lifestyle. You can incorporate different elements of Hygge in your living space and life. When you implement these elements in your lifestyle, you can bring out feelings of connection, comfort, and peace in your life.

Lighting

It is important to improve your lighting if you want to add some elements of Hygge to your living space. The use of soft and warm white light will create a comfortable and inviting space when compared to harsh and bright white bulbs. The bulb will be brighter if the bulb has more lumens. You can install a dimmer if you want to monitor the lighting in the space where you are living. One of the other things to do is to have floor lamps instead of overhead lighting. The latter will create light that will be too bright for the room. It can make the room seem a little institutional. When you use table and floor lamps, you can create a room that is intimate with the best lighting. You should also ensure that you light those areas where people relax, talk to each other, or read. Candles are the best part of following a hyggelig lifestyle. These candles create a soft and warm light that will leave you with a sense of comfort and relaxation. If an open-flamed candle creates a hazard for your living room because of children or pets, you can use LED lights.

Texture

Hygge is about using things that feel cozy and soft. You should incorporate accessories like pillows, blankets, rugs, and throws if you want to create a space that is inviting and warm. These soft textures will calm you down, especially when your anxiety runs very high. Soft textures will also allow you to give people some sense of safety. The way you decorate the living space will allow people to open up with each other. Any conversation you have with other people will feel more open and calmer in this space. Nobody will feel pressured or rushed.

Décor

You can create a calming environment by using different accessories like indoor plants, wood elements, and clean and simple décor. You should use these pieces, especially those that have a special meaning. You can keep pictures of friends, family, and loved ones on the mantel in your living room. You can also place some albums on the coffee table with some pictures of your experiences and travels that you may have shared with the people around you. Hygge is about connection and warmth, so you should use the décor to draw your friends and family in, and create conversation.

Warmth

You must understand that warmth is not only about the temperature in the room, but also a sense of emotional warmth. One of the best ways to lead a hyggelig lifestyle is to construct a fireplace. However, this is not an option for everybody. You can do anything that will create a warm, inviting space, and this will be a plus. Some examples are using candles, displays, accent lighting, and more. You can also use twinkly or fairy lights in some areas of your house if you want to create warmth. These alternate forms can be used as replacements for fireplaces.

Color

The colors you choose for the living room can help you set a cozy stage for yourself, friends, and family. It is best to choose some neutral colors like soft whites, whites, soft browns, and blushes. When you use neutral colors, you can calm your mind and create a calm atmosphere. These colors will fit into this style of living. The Hygge lifestyle is about creating a soft, comfortable, soothing, or calm atmosphere. In simple words, the Hygge lifestyle will promote an environment that is anti-anxiety for spending time with those you love.

People

As mentioned earlier, the Hygge lifestyle focuses only on building and maintaining meaningful connections with your loved ones. The objective is always to be present. When you nurture such relationships, you will allow yourself and the people around you to experience a sense of calm. When you are in an environment that you belong, you will feel emotionally secure. When you can maintain emotional safety, you can create a positive social experience. This will allow you to feel the benefit of calm, connection, and ease.

Activity

A hyggelig lifestyle will involve things that will help you feel cozy, connected, and peaceful. You will learn to connect with the people around you with ease. One of the best ways to do this is to spend time with friends and family. These gatherings are focused only on connections with the people around you and not only on the environment. You do not have to make it a black-tie affair. The Hygge lifestyle will only suggest the opposite. These gatherings will offer you to create a space that is inviting, casual, and also offers people space where they can focus on connecting with the people around them. This environment will allow them to feel comfortable. You can organize a game night with friends, family, or neighbors, host a book night, or invite people over for coffee or dinner.

Some Tips

Here are a few tips you can use to follow a hyggelig lifestyle.

Light Candles

Wiking says that you cannot follow a Hygge lifestyle if you do not have any candles. This is mentioned in the first chapter of the book. When you turn the lights down and light candles around your house, you can transform the atmosphere you are in with ease. To make this better, you can use scented candles that will bring tranquility to space. It is impossible for you not to enjoy the relaxing effects of the aroma or the glow of the flame. The smell and aroma are a big part of the Hygge lifestyle. If some scents or fragrances remind you of something wonderful when you felt comfortable and safe, it will smell like Hygge.

Never Deprive Yourself

You must ensure that you enjoy the little pleasures in your life. It also means that you need to indulge in whatever you feel like and that you are kind to yourself. The Danes are crazy about treats and other confectionaries like licorice and gummy bears. You must ensure that you do not focus only on eating healthy and always take the opportunity to indulge in those delights that you well-deserve.

Drink a Hot Cup of Tea

Have you always felt better after you sipped a hot cup of tea while you were wrapped in a cozy, warm blanket? If you did, then you should relish a cup of peppermint tea or any other flavored tea that you like. Wiking has an emergency Hygge list that ties into the joy of taking a break and the Hygge philosophy of comfort.

Unwind

Hygge does encourage you to spend time with the people you love. However, this does not mean that you should always have people around you. One of the best things about the Hygge lifestyle is that you should take a moment and pamper yourself. You can apply a facemask, repair your skin with the best moisturizing formula, or anything else that will help you unwind. You can also slather on some lotion, take a bath, or even paint your nails. You must appreciate this form of downtime if you want to follow the Hygge lifestyle.

Create a Playlist

The right tunes will always set the right mood. When you create a playlist that will complement your evening with your friends and family or evening by yourself, you can invite more positive vibes and coziness into the room. You can also destress your body easily. Install speakers and play the music you love.

Bring the Outdoors Inside

Danes hate sitting indoors during winter, so they love bringing the outdoors inside the house. They love everything that is made out of wood, including natural items like nuts, twigs, plants, and more. The smell of the fireplace and other wooden objects will make you feel closer to nature. These items are simple and stick to the concept of Hygge. You can find the right objects that will embody the outdoors with musk and other textured woods.

Keep a Book Handy

You also need to keep a book handy. This is an extremely important thing to do. After a long, hard day, it is better to get lost in the pages of a book. This book could be a biography, how-to-guide, or favorite novel. Make sure you pick a book that will put you at ease. Do not skim through the book since this will not be a very hyggelig thing to do. Let the story unfold and see where it goes. You should take everything in.

Unplug

For most people, their devices are their lifelines. When you put your phone down and turn off the computer, even if it is for an hour, you are doing yourself a favor. This may seem like a very difficult thing to do, but it will help you learn to be more present. You will learn to be more present in your space. This is an important thing about Hygge. Hygge will help you tell your mind when you are off duty.

Make Your Space Cozy

Big blankets and pillows are extremely necessary. This is especially true if you want to evoke a sense of warmth and create a comfortable environment. You can always make the environment cozier by adding more pillows and blankets. You can use calming ingredients like patchouli, chamomile, and lavender to improve the space. These fragrances will bring in a sense of security and peacefulness. It is essential to create a safe environment if you want to make your house more hyggelig.

Add Twinkly Lights

It is ideal to have twinkly lights at home. As mentioned earlier, the lighting is the best part of a Hygge lifestyle. These lights are festive and cheery, and they look great anywhere. You can use these lights in your living room, bedroom, or even on the patio.

Light a Fire

One of the best parts about the Danish culture is to huddle around the fire. This fire can either be indoors or outdoors. This is the perfect time for you to spend time with your friends, family, and loved ones. You should always be thankful for the company you keep. A fireplace will represent togetherness and warmth. This is the place where people will enjoy spending time with their loved ones.

Open Presents at the Right Time

This is a concept that you will find in many Hygge books. This is an extremely important concept to remember. It is always a good idea to open some special packages when you want to celebrate your goals or milestones. When you learn to appreciate these purchases, you will learn to link every item in your house with some happy memories.

Planning Hygge Factors in Every Room

When you redo your house, you will plan the décor in your room. When you did this, you probably did not pay too much attention to the emotional aspect of the décor. You also did not think about all the memories you would be creating in these rooms. Hygge will allow you to plan the elements in every room. For example, if you were worried about the wallpaper in your room when you were redoing the house, you would not have thought about how it would affect your morning routines or reading at night. You will soon learn to decorate your house so that you can make yourself and the people you love feel more at home.

Chapter 5: Why Are The Danes So Happy?

Hygge has become such an important part of Danish life that it is considered an integral part of the national DNA, a defining feature of their cultural identity. According to Meik Wiking, the CEO of the Happiness Research Institute in Copenhagen, "... what freedom is to Americans ... hygge is to Danes." This national dedication to hygge has been credited as one of the reasons why Denmark is always at the top of the list of the world's happiest countries on earth, in spite of their infamously miserable winters.

Denmark is famous for being the "happiest country in the world." It has a well-deserved reputation as a semi-socialist paradise where healthcare is free, the government pays for students to attend college, and the national pastime is cuddling in front of a roaring fire with a glass of red wine (or vodka) and a good book. Together, the Nordic countries (Denmark, Finland, Iceland, Norway, and Sweden) have ruled the world happiness rankings since the first World Happiness Report was issued in 2012, and the most recent year was no different.

In fact, despite the dreary weather, since 2012 all five of the Nordic countries have ranked in the top 10 on the happiness scale, which is based on six key criteria: freedom, generosity, health care, social support, income, and trust in governance. Denmark took the top spot from 2012 to 2014, then came in third behind Switzerland and Iceland in 2015. They then returned to the top in 2016 and finished second behind Norway in 2017. Still, having been ranked No. 1 in happiness for three of the past five years and placing second in the other two years isn't too shabby. And although the Danish Gross Domestic Product is only a fraction of that of the United States, Americans were ranked as the 14th happiest people on the planet in 2017.

In addition to their happiness ranking, the Legantham Prosperity Index ranked Norway, Sweden, and Denmark as the top three out of the 149 most prosperous countries for seven years in a row. The Legantham Prosperity Index bases its ranking on nine areas of potential success or failure including economic quality, business environment, governance, education, health, safety and security, personal freedom, social capital and the natural environment. Denmark, Norway, and Sweden also scored highly for education, entrepreneurship and opportunity, the economy, health, and social capital. Education and health care are a big part of spending in the annual Danish budget and Denmark also has some of the highest indicators of life expectancy in the world. Numerous polls have shown the Danes and Scandinavians in general to be the happiest people in Europe and numerous studies have shown that people who are happy also tend to be healthy and vice versa. As a result, more people in more nations are looking to unlock the potential hygge offers for increasing their own health and happiness.

For Scandinavian countries this trend is far from new, but hygge is now winning the hearts of men and women around the world. In Denmark there are special hygge-tours to parks, coffee houses, squares, and streets where you can go to make yourself feel happier. All over the world there are hygge bakeries, hygge cafes, and hygge shops with hygge wallpaper. Morely College in London has even offered a training course on hygge.

But hygge is more than wallpaper and candles. Hygge exists in our feelings. The physical things certainly add to the experience, but you can't make something hygge just by lighting a candle. Danes feel hygge the strongest when they're at home. Hygge is an incarnation of all those things that bring you happiness and a sense of comfort. Hygge makes you feel serene, content, and happy. It applies to interior design, our everyday experience, and our philosophy of life.

So why are all those stoic, LEGO-loving Danes so happy? Well, it seems to come down to the concept of hygge.

A Sense of Trust

Recent surveys say that a remarkable 79 percent of Danes say they trust most people. Not just other Danes, but most people. That is saying something. Personally, I consider myself a pretty trusting person, but that doesn't mean I trust more than three-quarters of the most people I meet on the street. And I don't think that makes me any different from most people. Rather than being seen as a positive, I feel like in the United States that level of trust would more likely get you labeled as gullible or an easy mark.

Okay, so where does the Danes' sense of trust come from? Well, the small population (fewer than 6 million) and cultural homogeneity surely has something to do with it. Clearly, it's easier to trust your family, your friend's family, or people you know than it is to trust someone you just met. But this seems to be an overly simplistic answer. The Danish sense of trust applies not just to individuals but extends across their society and even to their government officials. That's not something you're going to hear much of in the U.S.! In fact, many Danes don't even lock their cars or front doors, at least until it gets dark.

But trust itself is not something that happens on its own. As they say, trust builds trust. It must be learned and earned. It is taught through our everyday interactions in society and reinforced by trustworthy responses by those around you. According to research performed at Copenhagen University, immigrants from relatively low-trust countries who come to Denmark also begin to take on Danish levels of trust. And developing a sense of trust in those around you lowers your level of anxiety, relieving stress and opening up space for happiness.

A Functional Welfare State

The Danes place great importance on the equal treatment of all members of society, regardless of wealth or creed, and they resist the urge to place oneself above others. This emphasis on community rather than competition for personal gain is a fundamental feature of Danish society. At the same time, Denmark remains an individualist society, where opinions may be freely expressed and there also is a great respect for personal privacy. Outwardly, I describe my Scandinavian acquaintances as friendly but not outgoing, reserved but not cold. Unless you know them, they won't smile or say hello to you on the street and seem to make a special effort to avoid making eye contact or interacting with strangers. However, that is really just a cultural thing, not a measure of their true personalities. Once you are accepted into the group they are among the warmest, most caring people on the planet.

As has been widely publicized, Danes pay some of the highest income tax rates in the world— around 45 percent for an average person earning $43,000 annually and 52 percent for those earning above $67,000. That sounds like a lot, but they also get a lot in return: every Dane gets free health care, highly subsidized child care, generous unemployment benefits, and a free education from kindergarten through university. Actually, it's even better than that: College students earn a stipend of around $900 a month from the government.

Surveys show that most Danes say they gladly pay their taxes. According to Denmark's Happiness Research Institute, the reason Danes maintain such a strong social system is that they have come to believe that the state welfare model contributes to a collective sense of social well-being. So rather than seeing their taxes as a personal cost to themselves, they view it as an investment into a healthy society and a high quality of life.

As an example, because unemployment benefits are built into the system, losing a job in Denmark is not as big of an issue as it is in other countries. Known as the flexicurity model, employers in Denmark have more emotional freedom to fire or replace ineffective employees because there are programs in place to retrain them and help them find another job. Denmark also has a strong labor union presence, which provide a guaranteed safety net, with unemployment benefits available for up to two years, if necessary.

Additionally, Denmark has one of the most generous retirement systems in the world. Citizens over the age of 65 are provided for through a combination of state and private pension programs. And when you're not constantly worried about having enough money to live on you're going to feel much less anxious and more secure in retirement. In other words, you will be happier.

Less Time at Work and More Time with Family

The term "work-life balance" isn't just a buzzword in Denmark, it's a way of life. According to the Organization for Economic Cooperation and Development (OECD), Danish workers put in an average of 1,412 hours of work a year, which is the second-fewest hours of all industrialized countries. Spread out over all 52 weeks of the year, that equates to an average of only 27 hours a week. However, most Danish employers offer a minimum of five weeks of paid annual vacation, which brings the number up to around 33 hours a week. I don't know about you, but 33 hours a week still sounds like a pretty good deal to me.

Denmark also has one of the most generous parental leave policies in the world. The government requires all employers to offer up to 52 weeks (that's right: a full year) of leave — for either the mother or the father — with the government providing support for up to 32 weeks of this. And in spite of all this time off the Danish economy doesn't seem to suffer. According to the Organization for Economic Co-operation and Development's calculations of labor productivity (GDP per hour worked), Denmark ranks well above bigger economies like Germany, Japan, and the United States.

In Denmark you won't find a lot of people wasting time surfing the web while they are at work. The philosophy is that you're there to do your job and your employer gives you the tools to do it well. The idea is to work hard to get the job done and then go home. And in many modern companies the worker has the flexibility to work from home or the office and to choose their own schedule.

Children and Hygge

Children have a natural connection to hygge and Danish children are taught the value of being part of a community at an early age. They learn from those around them and begin to soak up the attitudes and behaviors of their parents, teachers, and those around them almost from the moment they are born. So, if their parents exhibit the spirit of hygge, the children are likely to build it into their lives as well.

Children experience the world with open eyes and when they are happy it shines through for everyone to see. Including hygge in a child's life can help them develop feelings of trust in those around them and encourages them to develop secure relationships with others. Reading a bedtime story, building a blanket fort in the living room, talking with them about their daily schoolwork, or even making a trip to the local park to try out the swings … these are all hyggelig moments.

No Bragging, Boasting, or Showing Off

There's an unwritten rule in Danish culture called Janteloven or "Jante's law," which is based on a popular satirical novel from the 1930s. The spirit of Janteloven is "Don't brag or show off. Everyone is equal, so don't act like you're smarter, richer, or better than anyone else." And they live up to their words. It has even been said that being average is the goal in Denmark. And although it has lost some of its grip in more cosmopolitan circles, Janteloven is still a big part of the lives of average Danes. People tend to dress informally (casual but not sloppy) and you don't see many wealthy Danes driving fancy cars or living in ostentatious houses. Such behavior is considered rude and unseemly.

Not only are there fewer outward signs of success or struggle, but failure in Denmark isn't a four-letter word. Because they have such a strong support system there isn't as much financial risk tied to keeping one's current job. The result is that people feel a greater freedom to try new things.

Danes Live Hygge-ly

Living a hygge lifestyle, surrounded by family and friends, is surely the key to Danes' happiness. People are kind and nice to both themselves and each other, which makes them happier. Hygge activities like sharing a meal with friends, reading the Sunday paper, or even playing with LEGOs (another Danish invention) help to eliminate stress and anxiety. Over time this leads to a feeling of comfort, contentment, and satisfaction with our place in the world.

Chapter 6: Instructions To Get Through A Miserable Winter

For a few, the winter is a magical season. For others like me, it's a gloomy, cold, darkness you need to hold up out. Yet, there's a superior method to get past winter. An outlook that includes embracing the one of a kind parts of the winter months. Enter the Danish idea of "hygge."

Hygge, which is an expression of Norwegian beginning, is articulated "hoogah" and freely means "comfort." But while comfort is a significant bit of the puzzle, hygge is extremely a greater amount of an attitude or mindset. As Natalie Van Deusen, teacher of Scandinavian Studies at the University of Alberta puts it:

"The best translation is comfort, yet not the physical comfort that you get when you put on a sweater or cuddle up with a cover. It's, even more, a state mental parity and mental health."

It's a feeling a large number of us feel when we return home for holidays. In any case, it doesn't have left when you head back to the real world. Furthermore, trust me, the Danish hear what they're saying. They have the absolute longest, harshest winters, yet they're perhaps the happiest countries in the world. Here are a few hints on how you can achieve hygge this winter and ideally appreciate it more than expected.

Double Down On Coziness

It may not be the genuine meaning of hygge, yet getting truly comfortable can, in any case, help. Fundamentally, I become a specialist at digging in at home and getting as agreeable as could be expected under the circumstances. Reading a book by the fire with a hot drink is hygge. So is eating natively constructed prepared merchandise while sitting in front of the TV under a pile of covers. You can never have enough blankets, pillows, warm socks, hot drinks, or cuddling with your pet or significant other.

To achieve a definitive comfortable environment, Susanne Nilsson, a teacher on the Danish language at Morley College, recommends you mind the space around you. It's ideal to avoid huge, void rooms, just as spaces that look cold. Dump the fluorescent lights and utilize different kinds of lighting to further your potential benefit to cause huge rooms to feel smaller and hotter. Meik Wiking, the writer of The Little Book of Hygge, suggests you light huge amounts of candles, use lights with warm, soft-lit bulbs, and get a fire moving in the fireplace if you have one. If not, even a TV with a phony fireplace video can help. It's everything about changing your home to coordinate the style of the period, so it feels like an impenetrable post of happiness and warmth.

Consider wintering your opportunity to rest and your warm home as your bear cavern. Blame the winter to do those things you've been putting off. Nestle up on the sofa lastly finish that book, remain under your spreads and get past that TV show everybody has been discussing, or hop in the shower and listen in to your backlog of podcasts. Do those things you won't possess energy for once the climate clears up, and you need to go outside. I've been investing more energy in my comfortable bed, tasting great coffee, reading books, and playing Vita games I haven't completed at this point.

Assemble With Good Company as regularly as possible

The winter regularly reduces the measure of time you go through with others. Harsh cool, foul climate, and risky streets make social affairs and outings an issue. But, friendship and friendliness are a fundamental part of hygge, and the Danish think keeping up strong social associations is useful for the soul.

There are two approaches to hygge-style get-togethers. To begin with, you can sort out normal, relaxed meetups with friends or family at somebody's home with snacks, treats, and delicious drinks. Helen Russell, the creator of The Year of Living Danishly: Uncovering the Secrets of the World's Happiest Country, recommends these social occasions are tied in with simply reveling and making some good memories. So welcome your friends over, have some cake, coffee, juice, doughnuts, or whatever you like, and simply spending time talking in your comfortable front room and appreciating each other's conversation. Often should you do this as much as possible? Star tip: break out the occasional things to truly embrace what the winter brings to the table. Lagers, treats, and whatever else that is selective to this season.

If you don't have a comfortable home, you can have hygge-style social events in comfortable cafés, bars, cafes, or even book shops. Try not to let those comfortable lounge chairs at the neighborhood café go to waste. My friends and I like prepackaged game cafes, where you can keep warm, have coffee, and play huge amounts of games for cheap. Furthermore, in case you're all alone in another spot, the Lonely Planet Guide to Copenhagen recommends hygge members don't need to be people, you know. Post up at a cozy cafe or bar and try to make some new friends.

Appreciate Winter Wonderlands in the Right Gear

I hate being cold and wet, so I don't care about going out in the day off the freezing wind. Also, thus, I've never put resources into good winter clothing. Might it be able to be that I detest being exposed to the harsh elements of reality basically because I've kept myself from being appropriately arranged for it? If I bought some decent winter garments, and they kept me warm, perhaps I'd appreciate it... Because it's freezing out doesn't mean you needn't bother with a little action, regardless of whether it's only a walk. Get a good coat, pair of gloves, boots, caps, snow pants, whatever you have to step outside, and feel 100% great. Once more, not "sufficiently warm," 100% agreeable.

What's more, when you do head outside, consider doing exercises you can do throughout the winter. It could be skiing, snowboarding, ice skating, sledding, or having a snowball fight. Try to value the exercises, sights, and sounds you can understand during this season, and you'll only experience during this time of year, and you'll stop wishing it was summer already.

Slow Down and Find Joy In the Little Things

Wiking summarizes the essence of hygge as "the quest for everyday happiness." It's utilizing the winter a long time to focus on the basic joys throughout everyday life, take a stab at relaxation and comfort, and seek after harmony consistently. At the point when you take a look at winter through a viewpoint like that, it feels a lot hotter. Who knows? You may even begin to miss winter come springtime.

Hygge Christmas!

Make a comfortable Hygge Christmas with our tips and lot s. Christmas is the ideal time to rehearse and appreciate Hygge!

Hygge (hoo-guh) is tied in with being content, comfortable, and getting a charge out of the simple and little things throughout everyday life. This Danish word and lifestyle are difficult to explain appropriately. It is best characterized by how you feel when you do something.

Hygge is tied in with being warm and comfortable. It is tied in with being with loved ones or alone. It is tied in with having a comfortable home and room, doing comfortable exercises, and simply getting a charge out of the basic things. Hygge is a method for getting things done and how you feel doing those things.

Christmas is the ideal time for Hygge. Since Christmas (ought to be) tied in with being with individuals, you love and like, great food and drink, comfortable indoor exercises, and feeling warm and content.

Such a significant number of the things that we as a whole love about Christmas are also so beloved of Hygge. This incorporates candles, genuine flames, warm sweaters, and hot soothing drinks.

Hygge is tied in with being warm inside when it is cold outside. It is tied in with appreciating food and drink that warms and fills us. It is about social occasions of individuals and enjoying simple pleasures and traditions.

Truly there is no closure to the Hygge you can make during the Christmas season. Winter is the absolute best time for Hygge, as it fits the feel of warm and comfortable that we feel inside when the climate is cold, and it is dark outside.

Here are a few recommendations for making a Hygge Christmas this year!

1. Candles and Lights

Candles and lights are so ideal for both Hygge and Christmas. They make a warm glow. Candles give off a glow and make your home smell dazzling. Lights put out a shine and liven up something dark.

Your Christmas tree is the ideal spot for lights. String lights all around your Christmas tree. There is nothing more excellent during the Christmas season than killing all your other house lights, and simply sitting taking a look at a lit Christmas tree.

Light candles on your mantelpiece, and your coffee table. Purchase candles that have the aromas of the period. These incorporate fragrances, for example, cinnamon, pine, cranberry, and berries.

Turn off your electric powered lights and appreciate the delicate shine of candles. They make an all the more smooth, comfortable light, rather than the brash electric lights.

2. Baking

Baking is the ideal thing for Hygge and Christmas. In addition to the fact that it is agreeable to prepare and spend time making something, it additionally makes your home smell pretty wonderful!

Preparing Christmas treats, for example, gingerbread treats, and more will put magnificent smells all-around you are home.

You can share your baking with your family and visitors. Any engaging is such a great amount of better with great food and drink.

Make baking a major piece of your Hygge Christmas.

3. Get the Outside

Nature is a major piece of Hygge. Nature is additionally so common all through the Christmas season. It is the one genuine season when we don't think twice about bringing a tree inside!

Having a Christmas tree is one of the most magnificent approaches to bring nature into your home. Taking a gander at nature and the outside makes calm thoughts and emotions in us.

If you feel awful about having a real Christmas tree – and truly there is nothing so uncommon as having that real tree up at Christmas time with its exceptional smell, consider purchasing a tree with a ball root so that you can replant it after Christmas.

Wreaths are additionally an awesome method for acquiring the outside. Spot a wreath on your front door, on your mantelpiece, and anyplace else in your home. You need some greenery. Wreaths are anything but difficult to make with only a couple of pine branches.

You can be as insignificant as you need to with including nature inside. Only a couple of pine branches in a vase on your table can instill a superb feeling of the outdoors and nature.

4. Make your Home Cozy and Comfortable

Hygge, and Christmas as well, are tied in with being cozy and comfortable.

Warm and comfortable blankets and pillows are ideal for scattering over seats and couches. Twist-up in a cover to sit in front of the TV on nights. Twist-up before the fireplace with a good book, enveloped by a warm, comfortable blanket.

Make your home look comfortable and welcoming to other people. Turn down the lights, light candles, give extraordinary food and drink.

Your house is the main spot for Hygge, so make it warm, comfortable, and welcoming.

5. Do Cozy Activities

Cozy activities that you do alone, or with friends, are ideal for Christmas Hygge. There are such a large number of extraordinary comfortable exercises to do at Christmas time, alone or with others.

Welcome friends over and play board games before a roaring fire. Drink thought about wine and ate Christmas treats!

Comfortable up in a warm blanket and watch Christmas movies on your couch. Lay on your couch, hung with a cover, and read an incredible book!

Preparing is an extraordinarily comfortable movement, as are DIY crafts and projects.

Christmas exercises, for example, working out your Christmas cards and wrapping gifts, are acceptable comfortable Hygge exercises. Light candles, switch on Christmas music and work out the entirety of your cards for loved ones. Wrap and label your gifts and appreciate the occasion.

6. Play some Music

Christmas music truly fits Hygge. Relaxing Christmas tunes, for example, Frank Sinatra and Bing Crosby, played out of sight, will truly add to that warm, comfortable Hygge Christmas feeling!

7. Wear Cozy Clothes

The clothes you wear are so imperative to feeling comfortable, warm, and content.

It is alright to wear your night robe the entire day if you need to while laying on the couch reading a book or watching a film!

Wear warm garments (however not smothering), agreeable, and that vibe great. Fleece sweaters, warm knitted socks, PJs, and workout pants are all alright!

Finding satisfaction busy working – the "Hygge Way."

Nick Marks, a specialist on health, states: "Individuals who are happier at work are more profitable, increasingly connected with, more imaginative, and have better concentration."

Being happy grinding away is quintessential as we will, in general, spend the better piece of our lives in the workplace.

This is the specific motivation behind why one should look for a calling that is certain to fulfill in the long-term.

You may be asking why we're mentioning this. Indeed, it turns out to work fulfillment has a great deal to do with the Scandinavian lifestyle and the hygge itself. And, this goes a long way past having some hygge-Esque plan components in your beginning up space.

Something beyond an insignificant plan thing, it's tied in with building up close to home space, having a sense of security, and motivated in the professional environment.

It is anything but an incident that the nations with hygge ingrained in their national DNA are also the ones with the absolute most liberal attitudes towards work plans.

Giving workers adequate measures of individual time and offering adaptability like this for increased profitability, Scandinavians, without a doubt, realize how to use hygge standards to the benefit of the enterprise.

Styling a hygge-Esque office

Leading – get the "right look."

Of course, we slammed the possibility of hygge being a shallow looks-just thing. And it truly isn't. The appearance does make a difference, as it assists with attaining the correct mentality.

Pick the correct shades

With regards to altering your office by hygge standards, it's about light tones – whites compared with beige and rosewood colors. Consolidating natural and mechanical, just as provincial and current moderate feel, is another quality that is quintessential to a genuine hygge experience.

By and by, this recommends the utilization of recovered wood, revamped furniture, and rough sawn elements. In certain respects, you may easily mistake hygge inside with natural stylistic layout style as both offer numerous comparative characteristics, depending heavily on clever mixes of natural and mechanical plan components.

The two styles, as often as possible, acquire components from one another and may even be utilized conversely or with regards to one another.

Keeping it warm with delicious beverages

If you love tea, espresso, or hot cocoa with some whipped cream and crushed spearmint candy sprinkled on top, at that point, you'll appreciate this part of hygge.

It's an obvious fact that an XXL-size mug with any of the referenced refreshments is a typical quality overall hygge-related imagery. The pattern has additionally found its way into the cutting edge office space.

Regardless of whether it's a central corporate command or a cooperating spot, bothering your path to the more elite classes isn't believable without a particular wooden table and a fuming cup of coffee resting on it.

Have some yummy snacks in your desk drawer

Where there's a cup of tasty drinks, will undoubtedly be a bowl of complementing snacks. Trust us, these simple, maybe even trite nuances make a major piece of a big motivator for hygge. Regardless of whether its home-made macaroons or a chocolate bar, having a delicious treat in an arm's span is the sort of a simple pleasure that makes the hygge magic work.

If you've at any point read one of the numerous hygge definitions, there's a once in a lifetime opportunity you saw a recurring pattern – the way of thinking firmly advocates being available.

Practically speaking, this means capitalizing on small-time delights. Read a book, record your thinking, thoughts, and keep an individual diary. Take frequent walks, change to bicycle as your essential methods for transportation.

Being in contact with nature around all of you, the while relaxing in your little world, are the foundations of care – definitive state of mind with regards to both understanding and getting a charge out of hygge.

Keep it innovative and individual

One of the most disregarded characteristics of hygge is the way that it opens space for immense creativity. Although certain tropes are basic to all hygge-motivated interiors, it doesn't mean you ought to blindly mirror the given an example without even the slightest bit of character. In short – there's no compelling reason to repeat an IKEA stock room look.

As such, explore, allow yourself little deviations from the subject, and, above everything, hush up about it genuine.

Motivational quotes or some other symbolism you partner with achievements will be an invite expansion to your office space.

For a more close to home interpretation of the subject, you should seriously mull over a lot of Polaroid photographs showed on a cork wall or pegged to a wire that extends over the entire office space. Then again, you should use chalkboard walls to design and overhaul your office space as per your state of mind.

Let the nature inside your office space

Utilize plants. The greater the amount of them, the better. Aside from being a pure visual treat and easily supplementing your office inside, plants give normal methods for filtering the air around you and combat environment-induced stress.

Music saves lives

Another fundamental piece of Hygge theory is an audial delight.

Great music is attempted and tried the device for those experiencing difficulty keeping up their core interest. Improving one's work process and filling in as a good stress-reliever, carefully chosen music, will give a calming score to your day.

Our recommendation — this specially curated Spotify playlist, featuring tracks that will guarantee pleasant vibes without making you feel too comfortable to deliver your assignments.

Warm light

This one is simple — since Hygge is generally about feeling warm and comfortable inside and outside, it just bodes well to go through warm tones to light your office. Aside from the standard lighting that you should use for proficient duties, you can make an extraordinary state of mind by utilizing scented candles and string lights.

Go the "Scandi Way"

Presently, we feel compelled to pressure this one as much as possible. However, mimicking Nordic gratefulness for light and spacious insides is the correct approach in case you're seeking after the reading material hygge look.

With simplicity, utility, and magnificence at the center, Scandinavian houses/condos have a pure style that focuses on clean lines, warmth, and elegance. Practically speaking, this implies a ton of whites and hearty muted tones.

While floors ought to ideally be wooden, couches and easy chairs are frequently decorated with throw pillows and snuggly covers. Another significant thing to remember — try to dial back on accessories. Packed structure with lots of conspicuous tones is the total inverse of the great hygge look.

Some extra rules

Surrender to little yet rewarding pleasures

Try not to go excessively hard on yourself and remember that life's excellence is to be looked for in the little things. As such — don't deny yourself of the seemingly insignificant details that calm your soul.

Had a long and hard day at work — have that one glass of red wine. Had a good exercise at the rec center — allow yourself that one bit of chocolate. Try not to deny yourself of the seemingly insignificant details that soothe your soul.

Have a tech-detox in any event once in seven days

Presently, this may be a significant request to our tech-accustomed age, yet a day-long tech chaste is known to take care of no doubt.

This, in any case, doesn't mean total isolation and a sudden communication breakdown among you and your people. An incredible opposite – welcome them to your place and appreciate a genuine, eye-to-eye discussion with them. Nothing superior to restricting your online presence and trading it for a night of shared talks and laughter.

Chapter 7: Turning Your Home Into A Hyggelig Home

Now that we have spent a little bit of time talking about Hygge and how you are able to add it into some of the different aspects of your current lifestyle, it is time to discuss how you are able to bring this whole idea into your home. The home is very important when it comes to Hygge; because it is an area where you will spend a lot of time, in between eating meals, relaxing, sleeping, and having guests over. You need to make sure that when you are at home, you feel completely comfortable. If you can't be comfortable in your own home, what chance do you have to feel comfortable anywhere else in your life? The design and the layout of your home will be really important in order to ensure that you are able to bring Hygge into it.

You do not need to have a lot of money or be an expert in interior design in order to make sure that your home fits this mold, but you do need to be very aware of the way that you are setting up your home if you would like to make sure that it is comfortable and will allow you to be yourself. You need to, above all, consider what is going to make you and your family, or anyone else who lives in the home, feel comfortable. There needs to be some purpose to your designing, but remember that what makes one family comfortable is not going to necessarily do the same for another family, which is why Danish homes can look different.

So, one of the things that you can consider when it comes to designing your hyggelig home is the color. Often, these homes are going to be in a simple color. Neutral colors do work well, but as long as it is kind of a simple color, without a lot of busy patterns that could be distracting, it will work in this kind of home as well. There isn't one look that goes with all of these homes, so pick out a color that you like and that will make you feel warm, comfortable, and relaxed when you are inside.

The price for decorating the home is not all that important either. You don't have to be rich to make your home feel comfortable and ready to sit back and relax. The idea of Hygge is mainly based on the middle class; so, there wasn't necessarily a lot of money to throw into the design of the home. Mostly, it is about knowing what will make you sit back and feel comfortable and at home, and then you work on the design from there.

As you can see, the things that will work in the home will vary for each family that is designing their home. Some people may like a little bit lighter color while others are going to go for the darker ones. The whole design, as well as the style that goes into one of these hyggelig homes, is going to vary a lot about your personal taste.

There are a few things that you are going to notice about a hyggelig home, though. First, most of them will have a fireplace of some sort. This is because the fireplace is really relaxing and inviting and can be one of the center points in the gatherings that you will have there. In addition, the price about items in the home is not that important. No one cares if you have a really expensive item or if you go for something that is a bit cheaper to go with your budget. While most Danes will save up the money to get the more expensive item if that is what they really want for their home, no one is going to judge if you pick a more expensive or less expensive item and put it in your home.

Don't feel too worried about how to decorate the home or about the styling of your hyggelig home. Basically, the only way that you are going to fail at creating one of these great homes is if you create an environment that you don't feel comfortable or at home with. So, go with some of your personal tastes, keep it simple, and you will be just fine.

Add some more lighting

Most Danish homes are going to make sure that the lighting they have in their homes will be cozy, warm, and pleasant. There are different ways that you will be able to do this, but keeping the harsh and bright lights out of your home is a complete must. Instead of going with these bright lights, the ones that will be hard in the eyes and show off all the different corners of the home, most Danish homes are going to go with soft lamps and other fairy lights that give off more of a yellow color inside of the house.

This does not mean that you can't have some brighter lights in the home. There are times when you need to get some work done in the home at night or when you are cooking when the brighter lights can be nice. What many families do for this is have a variety of lights around the home. They will keep quite a few lights around the home so that they can turn on a lot of them, and get brighter lighting when they need, but then they can turn them off and just rely on some of the darker lights when that works for them as well.

In terms of lighting, many Hyggelig homes are going to rely a lot on candles. The warmth and light that come from candles are often perfect for the intimate and nice conversations that you will have during these times, and you are going to just feel warm and cozy when you see some of these candles around. It is pretty common during a Hygge gathering to find candles all over the place to help set up the mood.

Add in more blankets and cushions

Another thing that you are able to add into your Hyggelig home is to add a lot of texture into the home with cushions and blankets. There is nothing that is as comfortable and relaxing as curling up on a sofa or a chair and wrapping yourself up in plenty of blankets to keep warm and toasty. In fact, many times the Danish people will curl up with a blanket to relax and feel better, even if they are not feeling cold.

There are many ways that you are able to add in some more blankets to your home. You can make some of your own, with the idea that we talked about in the previous chapter of knitting to give yourself some free time during the day. You can purchase some from the store to help bring some texture in as well. Some people enjoy getting ones that are handed down from family members over the years. There isn't really any way that is better than others when it comes to adding in more of the texture, but having nice thick blankets and cushions in the home can lead to the feeling of Hygge, and can make it more relaxed and open.

Declutter the home

If you have a home that is really cluttered, you will find that it is hard to feel like your home is hyggelig. You need to learn how to clean up some of that mess and keep the clutter away as much as possible. One of the best ways to be able to do this is to figure out how to get rid of as much of the stuff that is around you as possible.

For those who are worried that there just may be too much clutter around their homes and that they need to get some of it cleared up, should start right away if they would like to make their homes fit up with this. Go into each room and learn how to clear it up, getting rid of anything that you have double of, don't use, or is just taking up space. You can spread this out among a few days if you would like, but make sure to get as much of it cleared up and organized as possible so that all of this mess doesn't weigh on your mind and make you feel stressed.

Keep the heat up

Homes that are hyggelig are ones that feel comfortable and warm. This is why the temperature is often turned up in these homes. If you have a large group of people who are coming into the home to have one of these gatherings, it may not be necessary to turn up the heat because their body heat will do it for you, but if you are sitting at home with just a few people around you, you may want to consider keeping the heat a few degrees warmer than normal to help out with this part.

When we feel warm, we feel happy. We can feel comfortable with those who are around us, and we are more likely to feel content and like life is in order as it should. Adding a few degrees to the home, while wearing a blanket or having a fire going, can help us to get into the right state of mind that makes us feel good and ready to take on the world around us. Your home is supposed to be a sanctuary, a place where you can go to get away from the world and all the chaos that is around you, and when you make your home feel toasty and warm, you are helping to do this.

Put out your memories

One of the features that you are going to see inside of a hyggelig home is that there are a lot of memories that are all over the place. These families are not ashamed to have pictures of their memories all over the place, to show off to others who come into the home. This is not only a great way for you to sit back and remember some of the good memories that came your way over the years, but it can be very inviting to others who come into your home to be able to see some of these memories and see some of your past. Put up as many pictures and other memories as you would like all throughout the home and see how much hyggelig it feels.

Creating your own hyggelig home is going to take a bit of time, but making it feel personal, comfortable, and like you can really sit back and relax is the most important step. Each family is going to have some differences when it comes to their home, because there is just so much that you are able to do to make it fit their personal style. Adding in some of these suggestions, without even having to make major changes to the styling of the home, can help to make it more comfortable and homey for everyone who walks in.

Chapter 8: Ways To Live Hygge

If you want to live life with a Denish method Hygge style then you can get here some ideas. Here are a couple of ideas:

Snuggle

What activity could be cozier than cuddling? It joins pretty much all of the parts of hygge – comfort, unwinding, effortlessness, and investing energy with people you're close – in one. Snuggle under a cover with your pals, your kids, your dearest companion, your pet – or all of them meanwhile. It's warm and bubbly, and it costs nothing by any means.

Ride a Bike

Bikes are extremely well known in Denmark. Denmark.dk, the country's real site, says the capital city of Copenhagen is known for its cycling society and is perceived as the main official Bike City on the world. Bicycles are hygge because they move at a slower pace than cars, giving you an opportunity to appreciate the view. If you own a bike, think about cycling to work. Various examinations demonstrate that individuals who bike to work are both more beneficial and more joyful than individuals who drive. If you don't have one, check whether you can get one used. Destinations like Craigslist and eBay regularly have basic models in great condition for $100 or less. Another alternative is to join a bike sharing program, if your city has one.

Take a banner from the Danes and get in the seat. Visit Copenhagen and you'll see it isn't only a bike considerate city, it's a bicycle overwhelmed one. You'll see a more prominent number of bikes than vehicles in the inside, and the city is tied down by 350km of cycle ways and ways. How does cycling help up your hygge? It urges you to back off and take in your condition. "You can see and recognize people in different way when you're on a bicycle," says Jeppe Linnet, an anthropologist who takes a gander at hygge.

Reading a Book

Reading is a hygge movement because it's an approach to back off and confine yourself from the occupied, fast-paced present day world. You can up the hygge factor by twisting up on a lounge chair with your book and a cover, or in hotter climate, sitting outside to read under a tree.

Reading is good, it can calm your irritability, it not only allows you to increase your knowledge, but also adjust your mentality, you will feel very relaxed, compared to playing mobile phones, watching TV, it makes you feel more comfortable.

Offer a Meal

Home cooking is significantly more hyggelig than eating out, and it's doubly so if you share the feast with a couple of good companions. To make your supper party as hygge as possible, focus around comfort food as opposed to haute cooking. New and regular ingredients are great, but a wasteful decoration is unessential. Famous dishes for Danes incorporate pancakes, meatballs, and rich cakes, but you can serve whatever feels most encouraging to you — regardless of whether that is your mom's chicken soup or you're most loved apple crumble. If cooking for a group is more work than you can deal with, hold a potluck. That way, every one of your companions can bring their most loved comfortable dishes and offer them, which knocks up the hygge remainder even more.

Sing Songs

Having a chime in your home may seem like something straight out of the 1960s, but in Denmark, it's as yet a typical act. "The Book of Hygge" takes note of that numerous Danish families have duplicates of a folk songbook, and they sing from it to "affirm the ideas of simplicity, cheerfulness, reciprocity, community, and belonging."

Put on Comfy Clothes

There's no genuine method to feel amazingly great while wearing a matching suit. To get hygge, you need to change into something simple and pleasant. Warm sweaters and weaved socks are exemplary choices for wintertime since they keep you warm, which is essential to the hygge perspective. Two or three hyggebusker (sweats or distinctive pants you'd never wear straightforwardly) satisfy the outfit.

Light Some Candles

Ask any Danish person, and they'll reveal to you that the easiest method to make a hyggelig climate is with candles. Danes experience a bigger number of candles than some other country on earth – an incredible 13 pounds of flame wax per individual every year. They even utilize the expression "lyselukker," which signifies "somebody who puts out the candles," to refer to a spoilsport.

Luckily, it's easy to discover candles at deal costs. Stores like IKEA, Target, and Bed Bath and beyond, and Amazon convey vast sacks of no less than 100 tea lights for under $15. Simply try to use them securely: Don't put them on or close anything combustible, keep them far from pets and little youngsters, and never leave a burning candle unattended.

Candles are the ideal method for making a warm, comfortable air in any room. The Danes know this superior to anybody, as they burn an astounding 13 pounds of candle wax per head every year. That is more than anybody in Europe, and obviously, it's everything down to hygge.

There's something about a delicate, glimmering fire that takes advantage of our intuitive, and it's easy to end up lost in its delicate sparkle. They also offer a significantly more easing type of light than a cold, harsh light bulb. Why not go through a night with your friends and family under candlelight, watching a family most loved film or getting a charge out of a board game? Just try not to let the hygge atmosphere quiet you to sleep.

Go out for a walk

Danes love to walk. Walking in nature - far from the residue and contamination of lanes and vehicles - can help dispositions and decrease pressure. Studies have demonstrated that individuals who climb or walk in green zones will in general be more joyful than the individuals who don't. Going out for a stroll at a nearby park is a fantastic method to clear one's brain from the worries of the day, reempower and in the meantime, to enhance wellbeing.

In the process of walking, maybe you see a beautiful scenery, pick up the camera and shoot it, make a small photo album, enjoy it at a later time, forget the time, keep the simple, natural face, the breeze licks your face, The birds are screaming, the flowers are open, the fragrance is around, appreciate these wonderful scenery, and thank the gifts of nature.

Drink Something Hot

Hot drinks will also give you internal peace. Hot drinks like tea, coffee, hot chocolate. In a cold day, there is nothing to do without drinking hot drinks.

You drink refreshments for the length of the day, why exclude rich parts like free leaf tea, locally developed hot cocoa mix, and marshmallows, sun-aged iced home developed tea, and common item imbued water some segment of your experience?

After burning some hot water, just wait a few minutes and you can drink a pot of tea with hot water.

Keeping grandmother's teacup and saucer around your work zone will assist you with remembering less troublesome events and warm memories.

Watching the TV with Friends

Watching TV with Friends and Family will be also a part of hygge lifestyle. With your family member you can see any kind of movie and reality show. So that family bonding will also be developed as well as your internal peace also grow up in a hygge style.

Friends can come to your house and you can see a horror movie to light of in your TV room and you can enjoy the movie. It will be a great fun if you see it in this way.

Play Board Games

Playing board game will be a very hygge way to build up your happiness. Board game will give you great entertainment and it will be another way to hygge up in your happiness.

Adjust your lighting

Unforgiving fluorescents are not what you need when you're feeling focused; put resources into lights with warm, orangey light and spot them around the house. These little pools of brilliance are considerably more calming on the eyes, and so will better guide fixation – also assist you with unwinding in your own sparkling haven.

Light a Fire

Sitting by a start shooting when it's cold and wet outside is numerous individuals' concept of an ideal winter evening.

Presently an anthropologist guarantees that this affection for the hearth is profoundly instilled and borne out of development.

His examination has appeared sitting beside a log fire causes our circulatory strain to drop and abandons us feeling quieter.

The explanation behind the loosening up impact looks back to ancient occasions when Stone Age man associated around open-air fires and felt protected and warm while holding with companions, he asserts.

Early people would have related the glinting light, snapping sounds, warmth and particular scents of campfires with unwinding and fellowship.

Chapter 9: Essentials Of Hygge

Hygge is anything but another pattern in Denmark, and it is an extremely old Danish lifestyle. It depicts a nice feeling or atmosphere. Also, however, hygge has a place with Denmark. Numerous individuals of all countries live hygge unconsciously. The thing that matters is that Denmark has an exceptional name for it, and it is an enormous mouth! Having a word for it makes hygge a conscious and shared experience. Hygge is a piece of ordinary language in Denmark. It is utilized as the thing hygge, an adjective in hyggelig, and as an action word into hygge. The nearest word cousin of hygge is comfortable in English, gezellig in Dutch or gemütlich in German.

For reasons unknown, the word has, at last, made it over the Scandinavian fringes and made rock star status in different nations. In 2016 Hygge has become the

Oxford lexicon expression of the year. The Little Book of Hygge by Meik Wiking has become a success and is distributed in around 35 countries. And, against its unique essence of getting a charge out of basic pleasures that cost no or little money, hygge got marketed abroad. In Germany, for instance, you see the word wherever nowadays. In a commercial for lavish Perfumes or travels and you can discover even a magazine called Hygge with content around happiness.

Hygge, in its unique essence, has an extraordinarily positive effect factor on the prosperity and joy of the nation. Denmark, like other Scandinavian countries, has an internal focused life because of atmospheric conditions. Danes don't concentrate on the absence of something, yet take what they have and make the best out of it.

At the point when a companion and his mom kicked the bucket, both matured just

49 years of age; it was a reminder for Meik Wiking. Confronted with the impediment and vulnerability of life by death, he addressed himself to settle in his alright ish work or to seek after a higher reason and increasingly important life. To serve society and leave an impression after he is no more. So he chose to face the challenge and went out on a mission to discover why Denmark positions so great in worldwide happiness. An action which isn't exceptionally normal, quite insane, for somebody living in a country with high social security. He made sense of the hygge method for a living must be a key angle in the countries experiencing elevated levels of joy and happiness. Here, I summarize the principle segments of hygge for you.

What are the elements of Scandinavian hygge?

Prioritize time spent with family & friends

A foundation of the significance of hygge is togetherness. Indeed, even it is conceivable to cozy yourself up hyggelig under a cover with a warm cup of chocolate and a good book alone, for the full pith of hygge it needs others. Not a ton. Only one, two, or four individuals from your nearby friend network and family. 60% of Danes express the perfect number to experience hygge is three or four. A major group of individuals is generally not considered very hygge.

It is tied in with investing quality energy inside your clan, where you can be yourself, have a sense of security, associated, and adored how you are. So normally, the best spot to hygge is at home — a spot to feel cozy or geborgen as the Germans state. Geborgenheit is a feeling of warmth, well-being, and love givingmy family and home. There is no space for social anxiety and pressure to exhibit a specific image of yourself. Be your actual self. Hygge is the social time for thoughtful people, and outgoing individuals can take a rest from the active outward-focused life.

"We are social animals, and the significance of this is observed when one looks at the fulfillment individuals feel involved with their general fulfillment with life. The most significant social relationships are close relationships in which you experience things together with others, and experience being understood; where you share considerations and emotions, and both give and get support. In a single word: hygge." — Meik Wiking, The Little Book of Hygge: Danish Secrets to Happy Living.

Lights assume a fundamental job while making a warm and comfortable home

The long dark winter months have made Danes the perfectionists of lighting structure! In Danish homes, a few sources of light spread all through the space to make a hygge environment instead of one major light on the roof. The utilization of flashing candle-light is crucial, and Danes light a greater number of candles than some other nation in Europe. The unscented is performed over artificially scented ones, yet as I would like to think, a warm aroma of vanilla, cinnamon, or gingerbread helps in making a relaxing atmosphere and stimulates senses and memories. Other extraordinary sources of light for warm temperatures are fiber bulbs, dimmers, and light chains. Moreover, the exterior like balconies or gardens is decorated with light chains until around March.

Meik Wiking writes in his book: "The dependable guideline is the lower the temperature of the light, the more hygge. A camera streak is around 5,500 Kelvin (K), fluorescent cylinders are 5,000K, brilliant lights 3,000K, while night falls and wood and candle flames are about 1,800K. That is your hygge sweet spot."

This statement is additionally confirmed by Jenny Mustard, a style and way of life YouTube influencer from Sweden: "Ceiling lighting is the place hygge goes to kick the bucket."

Indulging in life's pleasures and treasures

Hygge allows you to enjoy the delights of existence without feeling guilty. Eating and drinking delicious winterly foods like cinnamon rolls or drinking hot cocoa, chai lattes, or a glass of alcohol. All that is a piece of hygge. Danes have a sweet tooth, however, the demonstration of getting a charge out of those delights in the organization of friends and family is absolutely a decent lifestyle Danes and I accept!

Gratefulness

Hygge is being thankful, aware of the present time and place and gratefulness, and enjoying the simple things of everyday life. Consistently is a little life. Overlooking time and stress is a characteristic result of hygge.

"Appreciation is something beyond a simple "thank you" when you get a blessing. It is tied in with remembering that you live at this moment, permitting yourself to concentrate on the minute and value the existence you lead, to concentrate on all that you do have, not what you don't." says Meik Wiking.

Relaxation

Hygge is about moderate living and relaxing. Furthermore, great music. Everyone knows the healing impacts of music. Music causes us to feel great and lifts our faculties. Certain melodies associate us with our past by activating memories. Music influences us as genuinely profound. Make your claims hygge playlists or look at some on Spotify like Indorshygge or Ren hygge.

While together, we can attempt to take care of our telephones and with it the pressure and requests from the world. It permits us to be consumed into the occasion completely, to center and tune in to the next, and associate all the more deeply while locks in. "Hygge is tied in with giving your dependable, stressed-out achiever adult a break. Relax. Only for a brief period. It is tied in with experiencing joy in basic joys and realizing that everything will be alright."

How we plan our homes can affect our prosperity. Simply taking a gander at pictures of the wonderful inside plan make individuals more joyful. The Scandinavian structure is moderate, clean, and uses heaps of normal material like wood or sheepskin.

However, consider the possibility that you need hygge at this moment. For moment hygge minutes, make your little hygge pack. That is any box where you put in things that will assist you in making you feel happy and relaxed.

What things to put in your Hygge Emergency kit

Your Hygge Emergency unit essentially expands after everything that causes you to feel incredible, and quick track you to that subtle hygge feeling. I've made mine with 20 of my preferred fundamentals to help give you a tad of motivation to make your own. It's a sacred place with individual things as tokens of upbeat minutes and thankfulness. Things to practice self-love and to make a positive climate right where you are. Whenever you need it. You can go with the seasons and change the substance of the box for spring, summer, autumn or wintertime.

•Your bucket list for the season to survey without fail

•Favorite magazine

- Number of closest companions, social help, to call and converse with

- Journal

- Your journal

- Gratitude diary loaded with minutes and things you are appreciative for in your life

- Bath soap

- hand crème

- face mask

- Warm socks, maybe handmade with love?

- Chocolate

- Candles

- A warm cozy blanket

- Favorite sweater

- Favorite books

- Tea

- Letters
- Postcards
- Notebook& pen
- Photos or foto album

Chapter 10: How To Live In Harmony And Accommodate Others With Little Daily Gesticulations

Living with harmony with others is quite difficult, particularly in a world loaded up with the struggle, disasters, and varying conclusions. You may battle to feel in a state of harmony with individuals near you and with society on the loose. Start by associating with companions, family, accomplices, and neighbors. Concentrate on managing any disharmony in your life in a liberal, empathetic way and offering back to individuals in your locale. Ensure you likewise keep up your very own feeling of amicability, as this will assist you with feeling in a state of harmony with others.

Method1: Connecting with Others

Take part in network occasions. Check the neighborhood network sheets for postings about occasions like a square gathering or a network carport deal. Volunteer at network occasions and give products or cash to neighborhood occasions. It can assist you with feeling increasingly associated with your neighbors.

Method 2 Collaborate with your neighbors.

 Contact individuals who live around you. Thump on their entryway and bring over prepared products. State "hi" to them in the city be benevolent and agreeable with your neighbors so you can construct a feeling of the network in the neighborhood.

You can likewise welcome your neighbors over for supper or a beverage to associate with them.

Offer to support your neighbors. If, for instance, you have an old neighbor, offer to assist them with yard work or a task like clearing out the gutters.

Step 3

Spend time with companions all the time. Invest energy with great companions so you can remain associated with them and not lose contact. Timetable standard hangs outs once every week or once per month with various companions. Put forth an attempt to keep your kinships alive and active.

For instance, you may plan a coffee date once every week with a companion. You may likewise have a month to month game evenings with a gathering of companions.

Make traditions with your companions. Attempt things like getting together on the commemorations of extraordinary occasions or taking a yearly excursion together.

Step 4

Invest quality energy with family. Attempt to cause the time you to go through with your family important and critical. Have standard family suppers or welcome your family finished. Plan an excursion with your family, particularly if it's been for a moment since you have all voyages together.

Regardless of whether you aren't very near your family, you can, in any case, attempt to associate with them on occasion. You may find that the additional time you go through with your family, the more agreeable around one another you will turn into.

Grasp your family's customs and attempt to make new ones. Sharing life occasions and recollecting shared minutes makes a feeling of having a place.

Step 5

Be defenseless and legit with loved ones. Open yourself up to your loved ones when you need them. Try not to conceal your sentiments or avoid offering your feelings to them. Rather, be powerless so you can feel increasingly bona fide and genuine around those near you.

For instance, in case you're having a harsh day, you may tell your companions, "Today was an awful day. I need some perking up" or "I'm not feeling incredible today; I need some help."

Step 6

Be liberal and minding to your accomplice or companion. The approach you're sentimental cooperation with deference and appreciation. Give them everyday consideration and affirmation. Tell them they are critical to you and that you esteem them.

You can do this by telling your accomplice routinely, "Thank you for all that you do" or "I welcome you."

Method 2

Conquering Differences and Disagreements

Abstain from hollering or yelling at others. Do whatever it takes not to get forceful or furious at others, as this will exacerbate the contradiction. Take a full breath and attempt to react to others in a balanced, quiet way.

If you are exceptionally disturbed, you can take a stab at venturing endlessly from the circumstance and returning when you are quiet and progressively loose.

Recognize the other individual's resentment and offer to discuss the circumstance somewhat later. Enable both of you to chill a little so you can have a progressively profitable talk that isn't overwhelmed by feeling.

2. Counter indignation with sympathy and compassion. Attempt to react to any disharmony in your existence with sympathy and tolerance. Instead of getting furious, consider how you can transcend the circumstance and discover an answer. Attempt to relate to other people and work with their deficiencies or issues, rather than attempting to transform them or make them see your place of view.

For instance, if you get in contention with a companion, consider how they may feel in the circumstance. Attempt to sympathize with their perspective and react to them with sympathy, as opposed to outrage.

Recollect that various occasions have various implications for various individuals. Attempt to comprehend what they are accustomed to by saying, "Assist me with seeing how you see this circumstance."

3. Be an attentive person. Keep in touch with the individual when they are talking, regardless of whether you don't concur with what they are stating. Keep your arms loose at your sides and turn your body towards them, so they realize you are focusing. Gesture and state "uh-huh" or "OK" to tell them you are listening.

Abstain from interfering with them when they are talking. Rather, sit tight for them to get done with talking. At that point, take a stab at rehashing what they said back to them, so they realize you heard them effectively.

For instance, you may state, "What I think you said is..." or "What I hear you state is...".

4. Be available to settle. Some of the time, things don't go your direction. You may need to discover shared conviction with somebody you don't concur with or let go of your pride and acknowledge a tradeoff. Consenting to a tradeoff may assist you with proceeding onward from the circumstance and not let the difference rattle you or into disharmony.

For instance, you may discover a trade-off with your accomplice where you split the family unit obligations, instead of contending about them. On the other hand, you may arrive at a trade-off with a collaborator where you cooperate on a task, instead of battle about the extend or go up against one another.

Bargain implies that the two gatherings surrender a smidgen to encourage getting some portion of what each gathering needs. Be set up to surrender a little with the goal that you can both be upbeat.

5. Acknowledge that you may not concur with everybody. A major piece of living in concordance with others perceives that you will most likely be unable to be companions with everybody you meet. You may have restricting thoughts or qualities, and it might be hard to discover a shared view. Be eager to acknowledge that you may need to settle on a truce with specific individuals in your life.

Because you don't concur with somebody or agree doesn't mean you can't even now have sympathy and compassion for them. You can, in any case, associated with individuals you don't concur with and discover a feeling of congruity with them.

Method 3: Offering Back to Others

1 Help a neighbor, companion, or relative out of luck. Show everyone around you that you care by offering them help when they need it. Help them without desire for reimbursement so you can feel liberally associated with them.

For instance, you may see a relative who is feeling sick or unwell. Bring nourishment for them if they are too wiped out to even consider cooking.

You can help your neighbor by attempting things like scooping snow for them or dealing with their pets while they are away on an excursion.

You can likewise invest energy with a companion managing an ongoing separation. Cheer them up by welcoming them out or by taking them on an exceptional companion date.

2. Volunteer at a neighborhood association. Look online for neighborhood associations and charities in your general vicinity that needs volunteers. Get a volunteer move at your neighborhood destitute asylum or women's safe house. Give your opportunity to a charity drive or at a neighborhood expressions celebration. Volunteering your time can assist you with a feeling positively associated with others.

Volunteering is, likewise, an incredible method to meet similar individuals and make new companions or associates. It can widen your interpersonal organization and make you feel less alone on the planet.

3. Give money to a noble purpose. You can likewise put your cash towards a reason you have faith in. Give a gift to a neighborhood support bunch in your general vicinity or to a national crusade that addresses your goals and values.

You may take a stab at giving cash to an admirable motivation once every year or once per month, given your salary.

4. Become a coach. Search for tutoring programs in your general vicinity at neighborhood network, or expressions focus. Check your neighborhood schools for tutoring programs where you work with children. Take a stab at coaching in a program like Big Brother, Big Sister, where you are combined with a youngster and go about as their mentor.

You can likewise coach others by being a volunteer guide at an after school program.

A few graduated class relationships at schools and colleges have mentorship programs for understudies to associate with experts in their field of intrigue.

5. Shop at neighborhood organizations. Offer back to your nearby economy by frequenting neighborhood organizations in your general vicinity. Search out nearby organizations and bolster them by going through your cash there. Become more acquainted with neighborhood merchants so you can feel in a state of harmony with your community.

For instance, you may shop at your neighborhood rancher's market and become more acquainted with the merchants who sell their products there.

Method 4: Keeping up Your Sense of Harmony

Keeping up Your Sense of Harmony

1. Discover a side interest or movement you appreciate. Set aside time to concentrate on a side interest that fulfills you, for example, painting, composing, perusing, or drawing. You may likewise do a game as a leisure activity, for example, ball, golf, or skiing. Perhaps you like observing terrible TV as a quieting, loosening up action.

Doing things you like to do can make you feel more settled. You will, at that point, radiate a positive vibe that others around you will get on.

2. Attempt yoga and profound relaxation. There is a condition come of harmony when your body and your breathing by taking a yoga class at your neighborhood yoga studio or rec center. You can likewise do profound breathing activities to assist you with remaining without a care in the world.

Profound breathing and yoga are additionally extraordinary for focusing your brain and feeling more content with yourself and your environment.

3-.Set aside effort for self-care. Self-care implies focusing on your needs and putting aside time to address them. You can rehearse self-care by scrubbing down at home or by taking a stab at cosmetics. You can likewise put aside time to peruse or snooze. Doing an exercise like going for a run or doing stretches can likewise act naturally care.

If you have an occupied, disorganized timetable, have a go at putting aside 30 minutes to one hour daily where you center around self-care. Timetable it in so you can't skip it or forget about it.

4. Utilize positive confirmations. Positive confirmations can assist you with moving toward your life and everyone around you with amicability and liberality. State positive insistences in the first part of the prior day, taking off for the afternoon or around evening time before bed.

For instance, you may state, "I am content with the world" or "I feel agreeable and cheerful today."

Attempt to live as indicated by your qualities. Exactly when your method for lifesavers up with your characteristics and feelings, you feel quieter as a rule.

Life resembles an ensemble, with high points and low points, numerous amazements, triumphal walks, and instruments in a state of harmony with one another.

So let me ask you - would you say you are happy with an amazing ensemble? Being in balance keeps up your bliss and prosperity as well as your physical wellbeing.

Having an agreeable existence resembles living as a woods does, where each component has a reason in this mammoth creature. Each part has a reason, and every one of the parts is associated with one another, contingent upon one another for endurance.

Here you have seven insider facts to carry on with an agreeable life:

1. Commend life - live with energy.

Your odds to be conceived were so minor and, yet, you are here. You have gotten the most lovely blessing there is - life!

Commend your life consistently. Live with enthusiasm and energy. Early morning you can get up in the start of the day and grin: Take a full breath and state, "It's another extraordinary day to be alive!" Pump up your motors, stroke your spirit, respect your body, give harmony, and quietness to your brain!

Is it true that it isn't just stunning to be you?!

2. Show gratitude and appreciation.

Like a stream encouraging the nature around it, indicating appreciation and gratefulness to your friends and family feeds your connections.

Tell them how significant and dear they are to you; how much better your life is for having them close.

Indeed, here and there, you may be quiet and consider the words you'd prefer to state - yet have no fearlessness to state them out of dread. The dread that, when the words are leaving your mouth, possibly your friends and family won't satisfy your norms, won't endeavor to be the phenomenal individuals they are.

Truly, it's actual, that may occur. Nevertheless, a great many people are perceiving the truth about your signal and invest much more energy.

Appreciation and gratefulness are your blessings to give as a byproduct of the considerable number of things you get.

3. Figure out how to impart.

If you have a pet, you realize that correspondence happens constantly. Your canine, for instance, doesn't utter a word to you, but then, you can nearly guess each other's thoughts. You see one another.

Numerous individuals whine that: "Our relationship is coming up short since we need correspondence. We don't convey." Listen, you are communicating something specific each minute when you are within sight of somebody; maybe you aren't imparting since you are occupied with accomplishing something different.

If your words don't talk in your voice, your body does. What's more, when you talk, the tone of your voice says more than your words.

4. Realize what you need.

Characterize what you need throughout everyday life. Know where you are proceeding to arm yourself with a well-structured arrangement on how to arrive. If you don't have the foggiest idea where to begin, start with the things that are absent from your life. What will give reason and significance to your reality?

Get inquisitive about the things you can accomplish and the amount more you can achieve. Advise yourself that, toward the finish of life, the most significant thing for an individual is the heritage she/he abandons.

5. Have empathy.

Having an amicable existence expects you to do a thing to the exclusion of everything else: have sympathy.

Have empathy for yourself as well as other people. Acknowledge individuals as they are, and tune in to discover new things, to comprehend, to truly observe the individual before you.

At times, the individual before you will be you. See yourself, recognize when life is extreme (for you) and give an embrace to your spirit. Excuse yourself when committing errors. Acknowledge your unchangeable impediments.

Once more, give an embrace to your spirit liberated from judgment, fault, or blame. You and everyone around you are just people.

6. Show others how to treat you.

How you treat yourself sets the models of what you anticipate from others. Approach yourself with deference. Talk pleasantly too, and about yourself. You are the watchman of what your identity is and who you need to turn into. Like a lion ensuring his realm, secure your prosperity, mental self-portrait, and future.

7. Remain positive.

Nearly everything that occurs in life has a positive part. Quest for that side of things and be certain that whatever life places before you, you'll discover your direction.

Realize that there is no issue without an answer. Look carefully and perceive what number of conceivable outcomes and openings are opened up for you.

Tidy up your condition of the antagonism (individuals and things) and focus, see and recognize the brilliant side of life.

Chapter 11: Hygge Formula: Happiness And Coziness Anywhere

"The man who makes everything that leads to happiness depends on himself, not on others, has adopted the best plan to live happily." Plato (427 BC - 347 BC).

According to the Royal Spanish Academy of Language, happiness is a "state of pleasant spiritual and physical satisfaction". This definition would fit quite well with Plato's version, since for the Greek philosopher, a student of Socrates; it lies in personal growth and is the result of satisfaction achieved through small achievements.

The Danish philosophy of happiness is now also very popular with us. The Collins dictionary- even recognized the term "hygge" as one of the most popular words of the year. Designers reflect the concept of warmth and coziness with natural materials. The internet is packed of style gears, blogs, and tutorials to assist "Hygge" to execute. However, the theory of Danish ethos remains a bit more complicated than a cozy sweater or a limited piece of designer furniture. So what is the real recipe for Danish hygge?

It is not difficult; you should put the cell phone away and switch off the television and the computer. Proceed to the canteen also to make a cup of tea, coffee, hot cocoa, or any other drink you like. Put on comfortable and comfortable clothes and get a warm, cozy blanket from the closet (in summer you can of course choose lighter fabrics). Light candles, make yourself comfortable on the sofa and just relax. Now think about what gives you the greatest joy.

When do you feel happiest? When you read books, meet friends or enjoy a family meal? On the other hand, do you love just to lie down and watch a good movie? Try to schedule a time to relax at least once a week. At the start, it can be difficult for you to find the time you need. However, think about how much time you invest in controlling your social networks, watch YouTube videos, or watch one of these TV shows that are repeated continuously. You will quickly realize that finding time to laze around with a cup of coffee and think about your life is easier than you think. Hygge stands for relaxation. However, hygge is also the ability to live in harmony and not to submit to the artificial demands and fashion trends of today.

COMPONENTS TO BE HAPPY

Meik Wiking, director of the Danish Happiness Research Institute, created the Hygge Manifesto, which describes all the ingredients in this delightful Danish happiness philosophy. These include atmosphere, warmth, comfort, harmony, joy, protection, relaxation, togetherness and gratitude.

A LIVABLE RESIDENCE FEELING FOR START

One of the essential elements of the Hygge philosophy is the warmth that a home offers. This refers not only to comfortable room temperature and comfort but also to the feeling of really being at home with people who are important to you. A home is a place where you can relax and be yourself. There is no need to bother about how you look or what you are wearing. Comfort comes first. A self-knitted sweater, warm wool socks, loose pants and a cozy blanket are enough to make you feel good. As soon as you slip into your Hygge clothing, you can make yourself comfortable with candlelight and a warm drink in your favourite corner.

"Do you still live, or are you still alive". This question comes from Denmark's neighbours but is just as popular there. Your apartment is your realm in which you can withdraw. You should feel comfortable at home - and this is relatively easy with a few tricks: candles, blankets, pillows, a fluffy carpet or a picture on the wall.

When it comes to hygge, light is of great importance. However, not every type of light counts, you should avoid artificial, too bright light. The best way to create a pleasant atmosphere is by candlelight. Statistics show that 85% of Danes use candles - an average citizen uses about 6 kg of candle wax a year. More than half of the Danes also say they light candles every day during the fall-winter season. Incidentally, scented candles are not suitable for hygge because the Danes find them too artificial. What matters is its warm light, as it is an antidote to the dark, rainy days.

Create an extraordinary place- a windowsill, an old armchair or an area with soft light and many pillows where you can sit with a book or a cup of tea for a quiet moment. You should be able to look outside so that you have some natural light at your hygge corner and can hear the storm or the rain. Bring a piece of nature into your house: leaves, branches, nuts, and a sheepskin. (This could also be the right yoga corner. You only need a yoga mat, some accessories, a statue of a yoga deity and candles. A nice bonus is a window with a view).

Ideas of arrangements at home in hygge way:

Make everything around you brings you well-being.

Leave only what is distinctive and necessary for you like memories of family, of a trip, your favourite books, drawings that have was made for you.

Create a stress-free atmosphere and bet on light colours, combine them with harmony and without great stridency.

Do not cram the spaces, so your mind will rest, and it will be easier to relax.

Wood and natural materials (wool, leather, linen, cotton)

Mix different textures to create warmth and a feeling of well-being.

The light

Unlike the Nordic countries, we do not lack light, bet on windows without curtains or look for ones that let the light pass and enjoy it even in the darkest days of winter.

Give warmth to the fire

If you are not chanced to have a fireplace, candles is also another option.

Do you know how many kilos of candles the Danes consume?

Not less than six kilos in a year

Take advantage, turn off lights and take out candles to enjoy a romantic and warm atmosphere. Of course, they are white and do not smell (as more unadorned better)

Enjoy solo moments

One thing that the Danes have clear is that we have to discover the pleasure of being alone, you can take a relaxing foam bath, make crafts, read a good book in your corner, listen to your favourite albums and for this, we have to create the ideal space.

Don't forget to socialize

We are social beings, who also need others to be 100% happy, have your home ready to meet friends and family, create a suitable climate for them to feel at ease.

Go outside.

At the minimum ray of sunshine, go out and enjoy your terrace, patio or garden balcony...

Turn these spaces into a special place to relax.

The sun and the outdoors will make you feel happier and at peace with the world.

Green, I Love You Green

It will help you create the environment hygiene some plant, bouquets on the tables

Taking care of them will also make you relax.

Do Nothing, Create Spaces for It

Well, that is an essential concept of all to enjoy without looking at the time, outside mobile phones, tablets and computers

Chapter 12: The Hygge Lifestyle

Hygge is about being happy, taking care of yourself, and enjoying life's simple joys. It is a way of life. It's about harmony, togetherness, simplicity, and contentment. Hygge is being happy and comfortable. It is sharing a meal with loved one. It is laughter, joy, gratitude, and contentment.

Spend A Few More Minutes in Bed

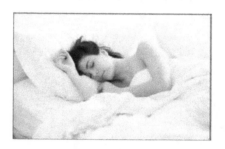

Many self-help experts would tell you to get up right after your alarm goes off. But, hygge is about being comfortable and enjoying the little things in life. So, don't be afraid to spend a few more minutes in bed.

Do Digital Detox Every Now And Then

Social media has taken over our lives and it's making a lot of us unhappy. So, to restore balance in your life, you have to go digital detox every now and then. Take a few days off from social media and enjoy the great outdoors.

Be present. Turn off your phone (or the TV) when you're having dinner with your loved ones so you can really have a great conversation with them.

Hug Your Loved Ones Often

Tomorrow is uncertain for us human beings, so hug your loved ones while you still can. Let them know how you feel about them and how they make you happy. Invite them into your home and cook delicious meals for them. Let them know how much you appreciate them.

Host a Potluck Dinner with Your Colleagues

You spend most of your waking hour with your colleagues, so make an effort to develop a strong, friendly relationship with them. Watch movie with them or host a potluck dinner at your place.

Read at Least One Book a Month

Warren Buffet reads at least 500 pages a day. Bill Gates reads 50 books a year and Mark Zuckerberg reads two books a month. It's quite obvious that ultra-successful people are great readers.

Reading doesn't only make you smarter; it also reduces stress and improves your concentration. It's also a great past time.

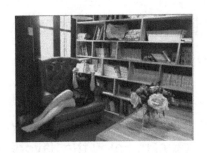

Do the Things That Make You Happy

Life is too short. Don't spend every waking hour in your office. Get a hobby. Do something you love. Spend time gardening, hiking, bike riding, writing, dancing, and painting. Do something that makes your heart sing.

Be a Good Team Player

Don't be arrogant. You can't achieve great things alone, no matter how good you are. So, learn to embrace teamwork.

Teamwork improves your patience. It also helps you teaches you to stay confident despite of your weakness and be humble despite of your achievements.

Don't Rush

You'll eventually feel anxious if you're always in a rush. Take things slow. Eat as slowly as you can. Enjoy the flavors of your food. Drink your coffee as slowly as you can.

Don't Work Too Hard

Hard work is great. It's the key to success. But, too much hard work can cause fatigue. So, take time to relax. Take a break when you need it.

Try Breakfast in Bed

There's nothing more romantic than having breakfast in bed. So, try eating breakfast in bed with your partner every now and then.

Avoid Stress When You Can

Stress is deadly. It can kill you, so avoid it when you can. Don't work too much and leave work on time.

Remember that when you're in your death bed, you won't think about those days when you stayed in the office. You'll think about the days you spent with your loved ones.

Chapter 13: Embrace Hygge Like Happy Norweigans

Norway was simply named the most joyful nation on the planet. For what reason would they say they are so darn upbeat and what precisely is hygge?

My enthusiasm for the word was crested in the wake of perusing the most recent World Happiness Report, a study of 155 nations, that was discharged simply a week ago.

Indeed, in spite of sub zero cold temperatures and long periods of dimness, the most joyful individuals on earth evidently live in Nordic nations.

As referenced, Norway hopped up three spots to guarantee the title of "world's most joyful nation" for the first run through. Denmark, the past champ for a long time straight dropped to second. These nations were trailed by Iceland,

Switzerland, Finland, Netherlands, Canada, New Zealand, Australia and Sweden.

On the off chance that you're pondering, the U.S. came in fourteenth spot, dropping down one spot from a year ago. Europe didn't passage so well either. Germany was positioned 16, the United Kingdom 19, France 31 and Italy 48. As anyone might expect, individuals in the Central African Republic are unhappiest with their lives, as indicated by the study, trailed by Burundi, Tanzania, Syria, and Rwanda.

At last, as in past years, Norwegian nations took most the top spots. Could the explanation they are so darn upbeat have to do with the Danish expression hygge?

In case you're from or have visited a Scandinavian nation, possibly you think about this clever word that is difficult to articulate. To give the signal, have a go at puckering your lips and focus on a throaty word somewhere close to hoo-gah and shade guh. Sort of like the start of the melody, Hooked on a Feeling. The uplifting news is, it's simpler to grasp hygge than to articulate.

Hygge is additionally hard to characterize, however is made an interpretation of freely into the English word comfort and is related with unwinding, extravagance, and appreciation. Be that as it may, Norwegians would most likely contend there's substantially more to the word. Hygge requires being available in a minute - regardless of whether it be straightforward, mitigating, or exceptional - that brings you comfort, happiness, or delight.

The word alludes to the capacity to appreciate the straightforward and beneficial things in existence with individuals you love. Hygge can depict delicate candlelight, comfort nourishments like a pork meal or home-made cinnamon cakes, sitting by the fire on a chilly night with fluffy socks, or basically being kinder to yourself as well as other people. It's tied in with transforming an evening cup of tea into an occasion with companions. A few people interpret the word as comfort of the spirit.

Along these lines, how about we return to the current year's bliss report and see what hygge has to do with the outcomes.

The report takes a gander at a few joy pointers, including a country's for each capita GDP (total national output, regularly used to gauge a nation's monetary development) social projects, future, opportunity, liberality, and debasement.

It ought to be noticed that in spite of the fact that individuals in Nordic nations are nearly wealthy monetarily, the report demonstrated that money doesn't rise to satisfaction. This is appeared by the amazing certainty that Costa Ricans are clearly more joyful than a lot wealthier Americans. Another financial powerhouse,

Japan positioned inadequately at 51. Mexicans and Guatemalans scored more joyful than the Japanese, despite the fact that they are a lot less fortunate.

Some would contend that Norwegians are better ready to value the little yet comforting things throughout everyday life - or hygge - on the grounds that they as of now have all their essential necessities set up. That incorporates free advanced degree, standardized savings, general social insurance, paid family leave, and at any rate a month of get-away time a year. With their fundamental needs met, Nordic nations can concentrate on their prosperity and what genuinely presents to them a superior personal satisfaction.

Perhaps that is valid, yet I figure we can take in a couple of exercises from the Norwegians and the manner in which they live.

Practicing hygge is persisted into their work just as recreational exercises. Staying at work longer than required and on ends of the week? Incomprehensible in Nordic nations! Most organizations shut down before 5:00 p.m. What's more, Norwegians have demonstrated to be less materialistic than different societies, acknowledging ease exercises and the more straightforward things throughout everyday life. At the end of the day, they center around encounters rather than stuff.

A solid accentuation is put on quality time and sharing dinners all together in a cozy environment. Need is given to keeping up valued connections and supporting their networks.

Truly, these nations have cruel climate, however these individuals are a healthy pack who show their thankfulness for nature and nature all year. In winter, most Norwegians aren't sitting in their homes all discouraged. They can be discovered skiing, hound sledding, snowboarding, snow-shoeing, and getting a charge out of the awesome Aurora Borealis. During summer months, they exploit the hotter climate to climb, swim, cycle, and sail.

At last, I think the report affirms that bliss has less to do with money and achievement and more to do with otherworldliness, our association with others, appreciation, a giving demeanor, and being available and careful.

Also, perhaps adding somewhat more hygge to our lives.

Along these lines, proceed. Eat that baked good righteous, welcome companions over for a glass of wine by the fire, or thrive in a candlelit shower. Enjoy the experience and let the warm, fluffy sentiments stream.

Understanding Danish Culture Three Things That Define the Danes

When moving to another nation, an expat will be faced by numerous new encounters and social contrasts. So as to acclimatize, it is generally useful to see a portion of these social contrasts. At the point when you begin to comprehend the Danish lifestyle, being an expat gets simpler. Here are hardly any bits of knowledge to help you along your way.

Life in Denmark depends on to a great extent on one idea - Jantelov-that everybody is equivalent and nobody is superior to any other individual. This idea was put on the map in the 1993 novel by Aksel Sandemose called "A Fugitive Crosses His Tracks".

Jantelov or Jante Law comprises of Ten Commandments that express that everybody in Denmark is equivalent, everybody ought to be dealt with the equivalent, everybody ought to conform and not stick out. The Danes still hold this idea to heart, so it is savvy to comprehend that idea. Attempting to be uncommon or to stand apart won't help charm you in Danish society.

Family life is significant in Danish society and family becomes before work or almost whatever else. This is reflected in the commonplace 37-hour week's worth of work, so guardians can get their youngsters from school and invest energy with them. Families still eat together and do heaps of exercises as a family.

Ladies have a truly adaptable maternity leave and just as men having the option to take fatherly leave after the introduction of their youngsters. Numerous guardians are away from their employments for 3 to a half year with no negative effect on their vocation or threatening vibe from their colleagues or organization. It is regular for work calendars to spin around the family life and not the a different way.

Kids are free to go with their folks to work; there are not very many spots where kids are not greet. The nation is alright for youngsters to play outside alone without supervision. Individuals are constantly stunned to see babies in child buggies dozing outside eateries, stores or homes while the guardians are inside shopping, eating or doing different things.

"Hygge" is another significant part of life in Denmark and you will hear the term utilized a great deal regarding social events.

Hygge isn't anything but difficult to make an interpretation of, yet the Danish to English word reference portrays it as "comfort, comfortable, merry environment, charming time". Hygge can be utilized as a descriptor, action word or thing.

The Danes love to "hygge" with loved ones. That generally comprises and lounging around drinking, eating, talking and appreciating each other's conversation and having loads of candles lit. Lighting candles in Denmark is a national fixation. The Danes love CANDLES! Indeed, even at work, individuals like to "hygge". The work environment should be a charming spot to be.

The term is additionally used to portray an individual's home. It is very "hyggelig" which means it is a "cozy and welcoming home". Individuals additionally state, "I made some "hyggelig" memories", signifying, "I had a good time". It is in every case better to state "Det var hyggelig" than "thank you for a pleasant time!".

You will before long understand that "hygge" is exceptionally difficult to depict, however you will know it when you experience it in a genuine Danish home.

How to hygge in the summer

It's anything but difficult to accept that it's about wooly socks and cups of steaming espresso before the fire, yet that couldn't possibly be more off-base. Hygge isn't carefully for winter – it's something that can be delighted in throughout the entire year.

You can hygge whenever of year and summer is the ideal season to make like a Scandinavian and get back in contact with nature.

A Danish summer is fundamentally the same as a British summer, with wonderful blue skies and light breezes combined with propping, stormy showers and sprinkle. Be that as it may, the Danes are a solid people, and a little downpour doesn't put a damper on the hygge.

The magnificence of summer hygge is that all as well as can be expected be delighted in for nothing – a fun day at the ocean side; a glass of wine in the nursery; perusing a book in the daylight.

Set aside the effort to connect every one of your detects and welcome the sights, sounds, scents and tastes of the long, languid days and mild evenings.

In the event that you need to channel some obvious Danish soul this late spring, you'll need to jump on your bicycle.

In 2016, bicycles dwarfed vehicles for the first run through in Copenhagen, with a great many individuals going on two wheels for driving and relaxation.

Jettison the vehicle and get some activity by investigating your neighborhood bike, and grasp the outside air and family fun.

In any case, as we as a whole know, we can't really depend on the climate. On the off chance that you don't extravagant an invigorating stroll in the mid year downpour, why not carry the outside in with some lovely crisp blossoms? Or then again take a stab at a Danish formula, for example, this mid year berry Danish twist, or their acclaimed smørrebrød (open sandwiches)?

Keep in mind, as Meik Wiking says in The Little Book of Hygge, hygge is 'the quest for ordinary satisfaction's – and that implies summer the same amount of as winter.

Hygge can't be forced, yet it can occur whenever, so sit back, unwind, and let the late spring hygge wash over you. Evaluate these mid year hygge tips.

Other summer tips for hygge

Natural product picking in the open country

Searching for shells on the sea shore

Welcoming your companions over for a grill and toast marshmallows

Beginning a vegetable fix

Riding your bicycle through the recreation center

Stargazing on a reasonable, warm night

Hygge may be new to my jargon yet the idea itself isn't new in any way—it's really a sixteenth century idea that has as of late advanced go into mainstream society. Not exclusively was it in the running for 2016's promise of the year, it's likewise an oft-talked about subject on our present marathon watching fixation, Ladies of London. So it's a great opportunity to get a curiously large toss and beginning arranging your best hygge life. We can help.

1. The Little Book of Hygge: Danish Secrets to Happy Living

You can't carry on with the hygge existence without finding out about the hygge life. As the title proposes, this New York Times smash hit is your manual for living like the Danish—probably the most joyful individuals on the planet. From showing you the specialty of candles and lights to how to fabricate better connections and take advantage of your "personal" time, creator Meik Wiking will show you the nuts and bolts of all things hygge.

2. Hygge Collection Soy Wax Candle

You can't accomplish full hygge without a quieting light. (Actually, "candles" is truly the principal section in The Little Book of Hygge.) Paddywax sells a full line of hygge candles, yet we're inclined toward the rosewood and patchouli fragrance in a become flushed clay pot with copper top—since candles need to look pretty and smell pleasant, as well.

3. Shag Puff Pillow

Regardless of whether you go velvet, shag, or cotton, more cushions = more hygge. Our current fave is this acrylic ivory pad from Anthropologie. The puffy cushion adds a touch of surface to a generally smooth love seat, and it'll match superbly with your...

4. Avoca Plaid Lambswool Throw Blanket

...plaid-designed toss! Like pads before the toss, you can stock your hygge house with velvet, cotton, or extravagant forms. Be that as it may, we'll cuddle up with this lambswool cover, ideal for nippy evenings at home with a cup of blistering cocoa.

BRB, we are going to set down for only a second...

5. Feline Study Mug

In the event that hygge were to be characterized by a creature, we're almost certain it would be a feline. What other creature consumes its time on earth twisting up on the love seat and washing in sun spots? So. Hygge. But since we can't really turn into a feline (as much as we'd prefer to rest away 90% of our lives), we can at any rate purchase the entirety of the feline item!. A hygge spot to begin? A feline mug for said above hot cocoa.

On to coordinations: Not just does this stone mug come in four cozy hues, it's dishwasher safe and Anthro sells coordinating dishes. Awww!

6. Philips Wake-Up Light

Awakening from a profound rest is so not hygge, which is the reason we're totally supportive of awakening normally with the sun. In the event that getting up at whatever point you need isn't likely to work out, at that point it's a great opportunity to put resources into a morning timer that awakens you semi-normally. The round clock reenacts the dawn and will progressively wake you up with regular light. You can likewise set up the clock so it bit by bit gets darker for sleep time. Hygge.

You can likewise choose from five characteristic sounds to wake you up with the light. While we're inclined toward delicate rings, yet you can likewise choose from seems like winged animals tweeting or a combo of both.

7. Cooper Lounge Chair

Regardless of whether your optimal hygge day incorporates perusing, marathon watching, or resting you need a comfortable, larger than usual lounger. Enter this Cooper Lounge Chair from Urban Outfitters. Without a doubt, the seat is fundamentally a redesign on your school residence bean pack, however it is much cooler. Simply picture it in an empty corner with string lights, candles, and a glass of red wine. Ahhhh. Hygge flawlessness.

8. Lit up Textured Stool

Use it as a stool or a side table or even as an extraordinary floor light, however whatever the utilization, simply realize that it's totes hygge. Being absolutely impeccable =/= hygge, which is the reason we're fixated on the odd points and finished fiberglass surface. It accompanies a bulb, however envision hurling in a dark light or something brilliant for a considerably cozier shine!

9. Beni Neutral Rug

Cold floors are so not hygge. Treat your toes with this handwoven New Zealand fleece that is too cozy as well as will add that exceptional something to your space. It comes in excess of twelve sizes so regardless of the room you're attempting to up the hygge, this territory carpet will work.

10. Send up a little prayer to heaven Wallpaper

This isn't your grandma's backdrop! Grasp an increasingly contemporary style like this group of stars propelled design from Anthro. Despite the fact that it comes in four hues, we recommend betting everything with the 12 PM blue. Rather than focusing on an out and out starry room, hurl this up on a solitary divider as a cranky emphasize. Saying goodnight will be considerably more hygge as you want for the star(ry backdrop).

11. Driven String Lights

A full-sized light is excessively brilliant for that hygge life, henceforth the delicate gleam of a morning timer and the unobtrusive light of the lit up stool. Instead of your conventional floor light, we favor petite string lights that give you the delicate sparkle without destroying your new hygge life. Ideally with an Edison bulb. Clearly.

A couple of better approaches to utilize string lights that are overly cozy: Hang them behind your bed as a fake headboard, hurl them in a container or container for a DIY table light, diagram a whole divider, or include clothespins and show your photographs.

12. Cozy Knot Pillow

Despite the fact that the DIY rendition is as of now making the rounds on Pinterest, we're apathetic, so we're simply going to purchase the ultra-adorable bunch cushion. This cutie cushion is pliable, comes in four lovable hues, and is the ideal complement for your rich understanding seat. Goodness, and the word cozy is actually in the name. You can't get any more hygge than that. (But, sewing your very own variant is really a super hygge action, so we're similarly as confounded as you are currently.)

13. Recoup Outlier Wireless Speaker

Lastly, the last component of your cozy life: music. This convenient speaker arrives in a stylish mint-shaded marble design and is Bluetooth perfect up to 50 feet with 8 hours of battery life. So whether you're investing energy with your tablet in bed or absorbing your air pocket shower, you'll have the option to hear your fave tunes from anyplace.

Chapter 14: How Can It Boost Productivity At Work?

Hygge translates into a workplace culture in which:

• Psychological health is accepted, for example, by developing safety networks by speaking partners

• Workers recognize they're "why"

• Leaders exercise mindful leadership

• Diversity of thought encouraged

• Everybody can bring their entire self to work

How could it advantage you at work?

The American Institute of Stress Reports:

• 40% of employees report their work as extremely stressful

- 25% of employees view their work as the number one stressor in their lives

- Job stress is more closely associated with health complaints than with financial or family problems

- An estimated one million employees are absent every day due to stress Whether you are the leader of an orga and anything that could potentially improve the happiness of employees and reduce stress needs to be worth a try, right?

But we're having that. You must be in a position to estimate ROI. And, unfortunately, formal research on the advantages of implementing Hygge at work has yet to be carried out.

With a little imagination, however, after implementing Hygge, you can find ways to measure success:

- Assess the number of sick days taken in a given period

• Assess the number of hours of daily productivity

• Assess employee happiness/well-being through quarterly employee surveys in which they self-rate on company motivation and commitment

6.1 How to incorporate it into your life

Having the work environment more hygienic is a great way to improve levels of employee satisfaction and engagement. When you're home, surrounded by fresh coffee, yummy food and laughter, cozy socks and Netflix, homemade cookies, and bright flowers, it's easy to maintain this attitude of convenience, well-being, and health. But often the workplace is where you need the most hygiene. You don't want to show up a nine-hour shift moping and feel drowsy due to lack of passion; you want to welcome your co-workers for the day ahead with grace and enthusiasm.

Work is the ideal place to practice the Danish attitude of this piece.

Here are some simple ways to make your workplace more hygge:

1. Philosophy of hygge: the working environment.

Some offices tend to line up with beige paint, fluorescent lighting, and chairs that are uncomfortable. Although remodeling your entire work environment is probably not feasible, you can start small. Provide alternative lighting such as lamps with natural light-emitting bulbs, or allow employees to bring their own if they prefer. Replace rigid chairs with more comfortable and ergonomic alternatives perhaps even some with cozy cushions.

Invite them to decorate it to their liking for those who have their own room. One thing everyone seems to agree on is that candles carry the hygge philosophy's highest degree. Most corporate offices do not allow real candles, but there are some great candles operated by batteries that imitate real flames. Consider offering them to your workers as a small hygge token.

They go as far as bright hygge socks in Denmark as workers enter the workplace. We're not going so far here at Beekeeper, but it doesn't sound like a bad idea for some of our rainy, foggy San Francisco days!

2. Eviting multitasking.

A large part of the hygge is currently living, which is difficult if you are constantly multitasking. Let's face it; we're all guilty of attempting to do too much at once. How often do you (and yourself) find colleagues reading emails while taking part in a conference call or listening to the story of a co-worker while filing reports?

Hygge suggests that there is no multitasking at all and that one task is taken into account. Which is a smart theory because multitasking experiments are costly and not practical. Urge your employees to turn off alerts that do not apply to them and allow them to relax and refocus for short breaks.

3. Hyggle your style of communication.

Hygge embodies harmony and unity on a more philosophical level, which goes hand in hand. Such values do not see work as a place to fight, but as a place to be more competitive and to work as a team to achieve goals.

Adopt an internal style of communication that facilitates relationship building with your colleagues. Celebrate large and small, job or personal achievements in the workplace and appreciate those for the company that go beyond and beyond. See how to integrate "sentiment analysis" into your internal communication approach as well.

4. Add more hygge to breaks for lunch.

Too many people are not taking a full break for lunch. Recent studies show that taking a break every hour increases productivity, yet when their team tries to enjoy their lunch break, many managers seem frustrated. Instead, management would rely on the full break of staff. Or try to organize more community lunches instead of team being on their own for lunch.

When workers have a serene place to enjoy their brief time away from work, it is even more beneficial. But if this is not possible, it can help to provide the right supplies for employees to enjoy a nice meal. Clean equipment and genuine utensils can make a big difference in the attitude of the team and can boost workplace hygge.

In a world full of chaos, it may be the best thing you can do for their happiness (and yours) to inspire your team to embrace the soothing hygge practice.

5. Bring a mug from home

It is comforting to have a freshly brewed hot drink to drink, even on summer days, and caffeine is a sure way to boost your energy and keep focused on your tasks.

"Take time with a colleague to enjoy a cup of coffee and discuss non-work-related topics," Gove and van Renswoude said. "Use a coffee mug in the office that you love." Drinking from your favorite mug is like having a piece of home with you. Don't worry about getting up for a refill from time to time, giving your brain a break from mundane tasks.

1. Creating a playlist of soothing work Music

It will be doing wonders for the mind. Make a playlist, including acoustic songs, with upbeat and relaxing tunes to get you through the working day. Wiking said in his book, "Apps such as iTunes and Spotify allow you to build an up and running hygge playlist. I'd go for something sluggish." 3. Spend lunch outside or take the time to relax when you're taking a break for lunch. Do not check your email, plan your next assignment, or look at your computer while eating your packed PB and J.

Get some fresh air if it's chilly outside. Walk around the block to the nearest deli or enjoy your packed lunch on a park bench, depending on where you work. Whatever is the case, getting outdoors will definitely help you relax for a while, and exploring the area might elevate your spirits.

2. Always decorate

have some kind of personal item decorating your room, from pictures of your family to a bouquet of tulips you bought on the farmer's market. Place string lights around your dressing room or stack plenty of tea on hand and old books around your office. Do not be afraid to differentiate yourself from the norm (in the policies of your business, of course).

"Instead of thinking about your office space as a functional, boring space, make it a comfortable, unique haven where you're motivated and efficient," Gove and van Renswoude said. "If candles are permitted, light a small unscented candle just for the glow and atmosphere at your desk." They also recommend making your office feel comfortable more like home with a comfortable chair, artwork, and personal items.

3. Hosting a potluck with co-workers

Comfort food is the root of all things hygge, and what better way to savor home cooked meals than to taste each other's dishes with your co-workers?

Eating together promotes hygiene time with your employees, it's a place where everyone can connect and be in the moment and enjoy being together "Alexander said". employees should organize a day of potluck instead of bringing lunch to themselves." When everyone shares, everyone gets hygge, "he said. 6. Do random acts of kindness to your colleagues Whether it's bringing a box of donuts to your employees. Sandahl suggests organizing more team-building activities to encourage collaboration, from scavenger hunts to tournaments. Gove and van Renswoude noted that once people are aware of hygge, they suddenly realize all the small, special moments in their lives. "Being aware of these moments allows you to create more of these moments.

6.2 Finding happiness at work – the "Hygge Way."

Satisfaction, for many of us, is a desired yet elusive term. Look around, and you'll see people running with an air of speed from one job to another. However, after closer examination, you will notice how they look stressed and unhappy. The more enormous scope of work, the scramble to reach deadlines and match teams, and quarter-on-quarter performance goals all decrease productivity levels and, unfortunately, lead many to flame out. Many of us wish we could just quit all this and retire in the hopes of finding peace in the mountains.

We know that we are not able to!

It becomes so crushing the burden of bills to pay, debts to kill, and so on that, we drop the blissful dream of early retirement like a hot potato!

Please! Not everything is lost. The good news is that right now we can find happiness here!

Once again, the recent World Happiness Report ranks Denmark among the top three happiest countries among the 155 surveyed, not once but for seven consecutive years. Resident Dane, Meik Wiking, was deeply immersed in researching the possible reasons for the happiness quotient that Danish people enjoy. He concluded that they appreciate a cultural structure called Hygge (pronounced hue-gah) among all aspects. In June 2017, the Oxford Dictionary added the word and referred to Hygge as social interactions of high quality.

Hygge is an atmosphere; rather than stuff, and it is an experience. It's about being with and being safe with the people we love. When we're shielded from the world and can let our guards down, it's a feeling of home. "Coziness of the soul," "art of building intimacy," "absence of frustration," "cozy fellowship," and "enjoying coffee together by the fireplace" are just a few of the phrases mentioned by Hygge.

Let's discuss the reasons why people in Denmark enjoy high levels of happiness, well-being, and a high quality of life, do we?

For some people, happiness seems to come quickly either through the natural optimistic disposition of one or through a set of seemingly serendipitous circumstances. Good luck takes work for the rest of us.

The concept of having to put effort into one's happiness might seem like a foreign concept. Shouldn't it just happen happiness? Everyone have moments in their lives that they are all in a place of happiness that has arrived so smoothly and softly that they have never acknowledged its arrival. Without much thought, perhaps we basked in its splendor. We embrace it just as it is, takes it as a matter of course, but that does not make it less remarkable. Yet joy is born for the rest of us from a series of conscious decisions and day-to-day activities to pursue one's bliss.

If you know it or not, you have worked your entire life for happiness. Sometimes the path, the determination, and the thoughts that led you there are not due to the joyful life that you are now living. Consider the education, job, and individuals in your life for a moment. Your past decisions and hard work now have a direct impact on (or lack) your happiness.

We were guided here by all our past decisions happy or unhappy. We can be led out by our future choices and actions.

It's about having a conducive atmosphere. Hygge can be indoors or outdoors. You may be bundled in one of our comfortable linen blankets on the couch with your favorite boxset, or in a local cafe with mood lighting, great views and staff happy to let you have a good cup of coffee when away for hours. Your hygge location might be a picturesque remote beach or a park bench where you can immerse yourself in nature and just watch the world go by at its regular pace.

Hygge decor Home furniture is a significant part of hygge. Think of candles (lots of candles!), fluffy rugs, slippers and pajamas, blankets, and cushions. We think our linen robes are magnificent to get the feeling of hygge so that you can lovingly wear them all day without the slightest bit of remorse. There is also plenty of texture and softness in linen bedding.

Share the hygge, or keep it to yourself, Hygge can be social, but if you choose, you can do everything by yourself. Good hygge can be provided by spending time with close friends, but that doesn't mean you have to throw a big, fancy dinner party. In a relaxed and informal atmosphere, a small, intimate gathering of close friends works wonders for inner bliss-remember to store up on candles!

When you're searching for your hygge, it helps slow things down and just enjoys the moment. It's living for now, whether you're in the bath, catching up with an old friend, or walking the dogs through a wood. Putting the TV remote and your phone in a drawer out of the way, as well as activities such as knitting, jigsawing, or reading, are useful ways to exercise sensitivity.

Hygge isn't seasonal; indeed, hygge is a winter thing for many people. The winter months are getting very cold and dark in Denmark, of course, so it's no surprise that the Danes like to make their home environment so cozy and inviting. But there's nothing to say in spring, summer or autumn that you can't hygge it up.

Don't overdo your hygge. We can't always exist in a hygge-like state of mind. If we did, we couldn't take care of all the day-to-day, sometimes stressful things that are part of life as well. It would be like a sort of hibernation to over-indulge in hygge, so nothing significant would ever be accomplished. Yet, of course, taking care of yourself is also very important, and we appreciate it all the more in the midst of madness by trying to get a little hygge every day or a few times a week.

Conclusion

Hygge is an interesting concept that everyone could benefit from applying to their daily life. It's not something that needs to take over your existence and you can start by embracing just a small part of it.

However, you'll find that once you start embracing hygge it will quickly spread to other parts of your life and become part of your lifestyle.

The basic principle of being present and enjoying the moment is one that everyone could benefit from. The fact that it costs nothing to get started makes it an easy lifestyle choice.

But the real benefit is in finding pleasure in the simplest of tasks. There no longer needs to be any task that should be considered a chore. Instead, even something as simple as putting the rubbish out can be an opportunity to enjoy fresh air, meet the neighbor, or perhaps simply enjoy a moonlit night.

There are plenty of books about hygge appearing on the market which can help to prepare you mentally and physically for your new lifestyle. But, the critical point to remember is that it's different for everyone.

After all, everyone deals with stress on a daily basis, learning to accept the beauty in small things can help to reduce stress levels. As previously mentioned this is beneficial on many different levels.

But, perhaps most interesting of all is the fact that hygge is already prescribed by doctors across the globe. While the word hygge is not currently used the principle is the same. Doctors everywhere tell people to take a step back, lower stress levels and focus on breathing and relaxation techniques. In principle, these are not so different from the techniques used when practicing hygge.

It may be a new trend in places but the principles have existed for years and will always remain a good way to approach life.

CPSIA information can be obtained
at www.ICGtesting.com
Printed in the USA
LVHW011937300721
693919LV00009B/494